Bio-Etheric Healing

OTHER TITLES FROM NEW FALCON PUBLICATIONS

Cosmic Trigger: Final Secret of the Illuminati
Prometheus Rising
    By Robert Anton Wilson
Undoing Yourself With Energized Meditation
The Tree of Lies: Become Who You Are
    By Christopher S. Hyatt, Ph.D.
Eight Lectures on Yoga
Gems From the Equinox
The Pathworkings of Aleister Crowley
    By Aleister Crowley
Info-Psychology
The Game of Life
    By Timothy Leary, Ph.D.
Aversion to Honor: A Tale of Sexual Harassment Within the Federal Government
    By Thomas R. Burns, Ph.D.
Condensed Chaos: An Introduction to Chaos Magick
    By Phil Hine
The Challenge of the New Millennium
    By Jerral Hicks, Ed.D.
The Complete Golden Dawn System of Magic
The Golden Dawn Tapes—Series I, II, and III
    By Israel Regardie
Buddhism and Jungian Psychology
    By J. Marvin Spiegelman, Ph.D.
Astrology & Consciousness: The Wheel of Light
    By Rio Olesky
Metaskills: The Spiritual Art of Therapy
    By Amy Mindell, Ph.D.
Beyond Duality: The Art of Transcendence
    By Laurence Galian
Soul Magic: Understanding Your Journey
    By Katherine Torres, Ph.D.
A Catholic Mother Looks At the Gay Child
    By Jesse Davis
A Soul's Journey: Whispers From the Light
    By Patricia Idol

And to get your free catalog of *all* of our titles, write to:

New Falcon Publications (Catalog Dept.)
1739 East Broadway Road, Suite 1-277
Tempe, Arizona 85282 U.S.A

And visit our website at **http://www.newfalcon.com**

BIO-ETHERIC HEALING
A Breakthrough In Alternative Therapies

by
Trudy Lanitis

*How You Can Use Thought Processes to Heal the
Physical Body Through the Subtle Energies of the Aura*

**Including channeled
material by:**
Kwan Yin
Lord Kuthumi
Edgar Cayce
Ignatious

NEW FALCON PUBLICATIONS
TEMPE, ARIZONA, U.S.A.

International Standard Book Number: 1-56184-139-0
Library of Congress Catalog Card Number: 98-87550

First Edition 1996
Second Revised (Falcon) Edition 1999

Illustrations by Trudy Lanitis
Cover art and book design by Melissa Gregory

The paper used in this publication meets the minimum requirements of the American National Standard for Permanence of Paper for Printed Library Materials Z39.48-1984

Address all inquiries to:
NEW FALCON PUBLICATIONS
1739 East Broadway Road Suite 1-277
Tempe, AZ 85282 U.S.A.
(or)
320 East Charleston Blvd. • Suite 204-286
Las Vegas, NV 89104 U.S.A.
website: http://www.newfalcon.com
email: info@newfalcon.com

DEDICATION & ACKNOWLEDGMENTS

This book is dedicated to my grandson, Griffin Gregory, who has taught me what the incredible gift of life is. He has opened up the door to a new vision and understanding of what we mortals are capable of experiencing. He has helped me to realize that there is a whole new dimension for the peoples of the world to explore. Thank you, my love! (With the love and support of Kwan Yin and Lord Kuthumi.)

Many thanks to those who have helped and guided me on this journey:

To my husband, Tony Lanitis, without whose practical suggestions and creative editing, this book would not exist. To my family, Philip Lanitis; Melissa and Alan Gregory, who believed in me.

To my friends, Don Crocker, BA; Pat Richter, MPA, CHES; John Echave; Anna Kertulla, Ph.D.; and Esther W. Radin, ACSW, CSW, for their encouragement and support.

To my associates, who attended my first workshops in Florida, Dennis R. Jacobs, D.Sc.; Judy Bacon, RDH; Carol Yancar, BA, BS, MA; and Ray Gaines. To Lorna Lynch, who provided space for my first workshops at "Wings of Light," her metaphysical center in St. Petersburg, Florida. To Dr. Paul Daniele, Director, Center for Metaphysical Studies in Clearwater, Florida for his support and the opportunity to teach at his center.

To my early spiritual awareness supporters, Jill Yolen, Trish Pfeiffer, Tacy Terzis, Dr. Lynn Harmon. To Dr. Garrett Oppenheim, for the study of past lives. To Dr. Samuel Schwartz, who directed me to spiritual healing via books and tapes. To Dr. Murray H. Kiok and Hilda Kahn, who made me aware of Radionics. To Dr. Patricia Heidt, who told me to keep notes on my experiences as "there is a book in there somewhere." To Connie Stardancer Hanham for connecting me with Kwan Yin through her "Magnified Healing" Workshop. To Jed Schwartz, Jin Shin Jyutsu Master, for his support and his teachings. To Anna Ivara, whose workshops on

"Healing and Creativity," and "Voice Dialogue," opened up my spiritual potential.

To my typing and computer helpers, Marie Beichert, Dottie Freeman, and Joanne Schwartz.

To my Spirit Guides, Kwan Yin, Lord Kuthumi, Ignatious, and Edgar Cayce, who encouraged me to write this book.

Many thanks to Lucis Publishing Company, New York, for permission to reprint two separate passages, one each from *Esoteric Healing,* by Alice A. Bailey, Copyright 1953, Lucis Publishing Company, New York; and *Esoteric Psychology, Volume II,* by Alice A. Bailey, Copyright 1970, Lucis Publishing Company, New York. These extracts may not be reprinted except by permission of the Lucis Trust, which holds copyright.

Many thanks to the C.W. Daniel Company, Ltd., Saffron Walden, Essex, England, for permission to reprint a passage from *Radionics and the Subtle Anatomy of Man,* by David V. Tansley, Copyright 1988, Health Science Press, Devon, England.

AUTHOR'S NOTE

This book is not intended as medical advice. Its intention is solely informational and educational. It is wise to consult a medical or health professional should the need for one be indicated. The information in this book lends itself to use by health professionals and also to self-help. However, the author and publisher cannot take the medical or legal responsibility of having the contents herein be considered as a prescription for everyone. While Bio-Etheric Healing may help some, it may not help others. Either you or your healing professional who examines and treats you, must take the responsibility for the uses made of this book.

TABLE OF CONTENTS

53

CASE HISTORIES IN BIO-ETHERIC HEALING

FOREWORD

Message from Kwan Yin, channeled May 16, 1994

It is within your power to be or become healthy. You can do this, if you have no hidden agenda. That is, if you do not have a subconscious desire or need for the illness. Ask yourself, what do I gain by being ill? Think fast — what are the advantages? What do I enjoy about it? Is it the attention I'm getting, or am I getting out of doing an onerous job? Do I *really* need to see the doctor? What is it a substitute for? What is it that I am kept from doing, and I have a good excuse for not doing? Think — the answer is important.

What are the disadvantages? Do they outweigh the advantages? You have to first decide that you *want* to get well, and we'll show you how! It is only when you are ready to commit yourself to true health, that true health will come to you. Most people rely heavily on what the doctor says. Many are seeking alternative medicines and healers, unaware of the healing potential within themselves.

It is this healing potential and its basic understanding which is your heritage and birthright that we are giving to you. You need not be afraid to trust it. It is based on sound principles and courageous experimentation on one's own body. Sometimes it is the only possibility one has for a particular healing. Always, it is the body, in its totality, healing itself. Occasionally you might use external medications as an assist for an interim period. The body is able to perform miracles, including creating the chemicals that it needs for healing, though it needs to be told what those chemicals are and told to produce them for itself. You need to supply that information to it! *And there are no side effects to such self-produced medication!*

You are embarking on a great adventure in healing work. You might even find it fun to see what incredible things it can do for you or your loved ones. We do suggest you get their permission first.

Approximately 99.9% of the healing occurs at the Etheric Body level and is the reason why healing done at that level is so powerful.

Kwan Yin, channeled March 18, 1995:

Kwan Yin, the goddess of mercy and healing for this planet, decided to help Trudy Lanitis when she realized the enormous potential in the healing work that Trudy had developed to help her own healing of a very debilitating rheumatoid arthritis. Trudy is a very gifted, creative person, who had the courage to do what no other person to date has been able to do in the field of healing. She has, in a very practical way, made the gift of healing available to humanity in the most effective and simple way of healing yet discovered and she is sharing it with the world. I salute her creativity, ingenuity and her selflessness. She is truly a gift to mankind.

PROLOGUE

In October, 1993, I was invited by a friend to a healing workshop on Magnified Healing, conducted by Connie Stardancer Hanham. This is a method of healing previously channeled by Kwan Yin to Kathryn Anderson and Gisele King. I attended the workshop and enjoyed it very much. During the course of this workshop, Kwan Yin channeled the information that those who were invited there had been "Ascended Masters at the Higher Realms." Most of the attendees, including myself, had no foreknowledge of this information and were quite surprised.

Kwan Yin was at the workshop, in spirit, guiding us through the steps of Magnified Healing. She wanted to spread its knowledge to a wider audience. We were told that this healing method is used at the Higher Realms with great success. Magnified Healing is effective on the Earth Plane as well. Shortly after the workshop, Kwan Yin started channeling to me directly. She asked if I would consider holding healing workshops to help spread that knowledge to a new audience. I told her that I was reluctant to do so as I was developing a new way of healing on my own. I told her I would feel more comfortable doing workshops based on my own work. And, in fact, I was not yet ready to do that either.

Once Kwan Yin became aware of my work in healing, she started to guide me to become more effective. In the early part of 1994, she asked me to write a book on my new concept, Bio-Etheric Healing. I had never written a book before, and since I am a visual artist, I felt much less comfortable with verbal communication. Also, I do not type and I am not computer literate. I have written this book longhand, despite some disfigurement of my hands which is a remnant of my bout with rheumatoid arthritis.

Kwan Yin has guided me through this work, saying, "it would be a boon to mankind." I wish to thank Kwan Yin formally for her faith in me and my work and for her collaboration and suggestions for healing possibilities. These suggestions went beyond what I had been able to develop on my own. Her guidance broadened the scope of what Bio-Etheric Healing is able to do, and made the results more immediate.

I began to wonder if Bio-Etheric Healing might be helpful with the terrible scourge of the HIV virus. I asked for information about the illness, and received encouragement from Kwan Yin to work with HIV-positive individuals. Her assistant, Ignatious, then channeled information for me to begin working with the HIV virus. He told me that the HIV virus was not a true virus, but is a lower biological form and is under the control of Pan, God of Nature and the Devic Kingdom. (See Chapter VI.) It is only through working with the Deva of the HIV virus that makes it possible to remove the virus out of a person's body.

He also told me that it was necessary to work with the Etheric Body as well. It is necessary to tell the Etheric Body of the person involved to heal and strengthen the immune system. He also said that clearing the Chakra System was important, especially the first and second chakras, and that sometimes the whole field of chakras is in need of healing.

I must admit, it seemed to me such an overwhelming task to deal with the major problem of the HIV virus. I did not know how I could handle it. Yet, I had asked for this information and now it was available to me. Would it work? Even if I succeeded, would anybody believe me? Would there be others to help?

I started offering workshops in St. Petersburg, Florida, in January, 1995, to bring the concept and practice of Bio-Etheric Healing to healing professionals interested in working with HIV-positive clients. These workshops began a year after I started writing this book. The workshops are ongoing, but will broaden in scope to teach the basic concept and method of Bio-Etheric Healing in the general practice of healing (including the HIV virus).

The specific purpose of these workshops is to recruit and empower a cadre of healing professionals to use the Bio-Etheric Healing method in their work where appropriate, as well as making it available to interested individuals. Workshops are planned for various locations throughout the United States. This work has begun and a cadre group is being formed. My book is written to serve as a "how to" manual and resource for them and for all other healers or interested individuals. This information also lends itself to self-help. However, it is not offered as a substitute for medical advice and may not be useful for everyone.

Kwan Yin, the Goddess of Mercy and Healing for this Planet, has urged me to share my work with the world. She calls it a great gift to humanity. She would like to see this book translated into other languages so that anyone who can read can benefit from it. I feel very honored that Kwan Yin has taken such an interest in my work, and has chosen to encourage and support my efforts. It is Kwan Yin's encouragement and help that has made this book a reality. I am pleased to share my experiences and to help the people of the world.

I feel grateful for Kwan Yin's love, affection, and prodding to get this book written and to do all that has been necessary to get this book out to the public. She has helped me greatly, as well as channeled many of the healings included in the book.

I want to thank Kwan Yin, Lord Kuthumi, and Lord of the World, Sanat Kumara for their encouragement.

Trudy Lanitis
Kingston, New York
December, 1994

Chapter I

BIO-ETHERIC HEALING
What It Is And How It Came To Be

I wrote this book to share the results of my many years of self-healing and research. This work has resulted in a new, breakthrough method of healing which I have named Bio-Etheric Healing. This chapter provides an overview, brief but complete, of what this new, breakthrough method of healing is. However, to understand more fully what this new healing method really means in terms of its exciting possibilities, it is important to know how it evolved and came to be.

Bio-Etheric Healing uses some of the principles of Radionics, but carries them much further in new and different ways. I first heard about Radionics from an acquaintance who lives in San Diego, California, where she worked with a Radionics practitioner. The woman raved about the possibilities of Radionics, and the wonderful things it could do. She also suggested three books I might read on the subject, the only three available in the bookstores at that time. I read them and I was hooked. I really wanted to try Radionics, but the logistics at that time of working with someone at the other side of the country from Kingston, New York, where I lived, seemed impossible.

Radionics was discovered in California in 1849 and flourished in this country until the 1920's, when some practitioners were jailed and others discredited due to the efforts of certain groups. However, Radionics was embraced in England where it prospered. Continuous research has carried the movement forward to the present.

Radionics involves healing the total person which includes the "subtle anatomy" of Man, the Aura, the Chakra System, as well as the Physical Body. The theory is that all disease starts in the Aura. Therefore, the best way to heal disease is to heal it through the

Aura, specifically, the first layer of the Aura, the Etheric Body. Radionics practitioners developed a series of instruments for the healing which could also be used for healing at a distance and for diagnostic purposes. They were able to claim remarkable things such as healing people in a very short time, and even treating animals and fields of grain and other crops, as long as they knew what the antidote for the problem was.

Radionics involves very intricate procedures and technology. It uses all kinds of complex charts and abstract symbols, as well as a variety of specialized instrumentation and even color codes to reach its patients with healing messages.

I reasoned that since I have a body and I can, and do, communicate with it for healing purposes using kinesiology, why can't I communicate *directly* with my own Etheric Body also?

The experiments began. I started by using thought processes to communicate with my Etheric Body. I would tell my Etheric Body to do some simple healings, such as work with headaches or with a cold, and to my surprise, my Etheric Body did it! An early example is my dry eye syndrome. I asked my Etheric Body to lubricate my eyes and, it worked! The dryness problems disappeared.

As startling as this discovery of direct communication was, I believe the real breakthrough came after working with thought processes for some time, when I realized that I was getting a *voice response* on a thought level. I was actually talking directly to my Etheric Body. It was helping me with its healing energies, the energies of my own body, to meet and overcome some of the constant challenges to my physical health. What an extreme thrill! And what a wonderful mechanism for self-help!

As I continued this work of direct communication with my Etheric Body, I made a new magical discovery. The Etheric Body had an active interest in the health of the Physical Body and was eager to help maintain that health and even to help heal problems when needed. This discovery of the Etheric Body's active interest was confirmed in later communication work with the Etheric Body of others as well.

However, though it had the desire, and often the knowledge of what may be wrong, the Etheric Body did not initiate any healing procedures on its own. It seemed to need direction as to what to do, and a request to do it, before taking action. I also discovered that this request had to be made with a feeling of compassionate ✳

love and in the complete absence of negativity in order to be acted upon.

All these wonderful experiences were integrated and became the conceptual foundation of Bio-Etheric Healing. I needed to test it all further in real terms with myself and later with others. This was all very exciting to me. I had previously contracted Lyme disease, which was followed by rheumatoid arthritis. I was very weak and ill. My knees eventually became so disabled that I required a cane to walk. At times, I needed a wheelchair, pushed by my husband, in order to get around. I was desperate, so I thought, "This is my own body, all of it, Aura, Chakras, immune system. What if I asked my Etheric Body to help me in this fight to heal myself? What would happen?"

And so, my journey of discovery intensified. Sometimes it was a little scary because I was my own guinea pig, moving around on an unknown landscape, but it has all been a wonderful experience — an amazing odyssey whose results have been well worth the effort. This book is the culmination of my research and study along this fantastic journey that has led to my discovery of an entirely new way of healing which I labeled Bio-Etheric Healing.

Bio-Etheric Healing is a simple and effective healing technique that is noninvasive, requires no mechanical devices or technology, and uses no drugs. Bio-Etheric Healing uses thought processes to direct the body's own energy field to do the healing.

The use of thought processes to communicate with the Etheric Body opens up the field of healing in a totally new way. This includes the possibility of healing problems that have had no previous history of success. Also, it holds promise for problems that now require drugs, which may be helped without the use of drugs. This opportunity exists because the body is capable of producing many of the chemicals used in healing, in the amounts the body needs. The body can now be asked to produce the chemicals it needs for healing and it may do so and, at the same time, do so without the possible danger or toxicity of overdosage.

I have experienced this many times, personally. When told by my dentist that I needed collagen for my tooth or I was in danger of losing it, I asked my Etheric Body to produce collagen for me. The tooth got stronger and was saved. In dealing with my rheumatoid arthritis, my trusty helper, my Etheric Body, responded by producing hyaluronic acid and synovial fluid to help lubricate the tightness and grinding feeling in my joints. The relief was almost immediate. Also, I was able to completely overcome a thyroid deficiency due to a partial thyroidectomy which left me dependent on thyroid medication. I no longer need to take a thyroid supplement.

When working with a client, a Bio-Etheric Healing professional can use this method to communicate with that person's Etheric Body using thought processes. Therefore the actual healing work is not limited to face-to-face physical proximity. Rather, Bio-Etheric Healing via thought process communication can be accomplished over great distances. I have also had this wonderful experience, helping family members and friends with their physical problems in places as far away as Dallas, Texas; Portland, Oregon; and even a truck driver en route along the West Coast. This is possible because, as Alice Bailey said, "The Etheric Web goes round the world, and everything or everyone that has energy has a connection and is enveloped by this Etheric matter."

At this stage, Bio-Etheric Healing seems to offer the possibility of helping in many of the body's problems. Of course, as there is yet limited experience in its use, some additional limitations may surface in time. It is not for everyone, nor is it possible for it to be useful in all conditions. However, the promise of Bio-Etheric Healing is great and because of its simplicity and versatility, it has the potential to influence healing all over the world.

This book was written as a "How to" manual to promote the understanding of this new method, its practical use and its application by healing professionals and spiritually gifted individuals. Also, this format lends itself well to self-help. The book will form the foundation of training workshops and will also serve as a basic resource and reference for practitioners.

"**All illness is rooted in the Etheric Body. When you destroy the root, the flower is sure to follow.**"

Chapter II

BIO-ETHERIC HEALING
How It Works

AN OVERVIEW

Bio-Etheric Healing is an innovative method of alternative healing which uses a set of Communication Skills based on thought processes to direct our Etheric Body, and through it, our full energy field (our Aura) to help in healing work. It is possible to have this communication directly with one's own energy field. Also, when working with a client, a Bio-Etheric Healing professional can use this method to mobilize the client's own energy field to help in his healing. The actual healing work is not limited to face-to-face physical proximity. Rather, Bio-Etheric Healing via thought process communication can be accomplished over great distances.

This communication, and the healing work itself, is possible because of the energy field which surrounds our bodies, and indeed surrounds everyone and everything on this planet. It is called the Auric Field, and our own individual envelope of this energy which surrounds our bodies is called our Aura. The first layer of our Aura, closest to our Physical Bodies, is the Etheric Layer, and it plays a major role in Bio-Etheric Healing.

In almost all cases, the actual healing itself begins at the Etheric Body level. It is primarily with the Etheric Body that we communicate with thought messages to provide it the directions for healing. It is in a sense the "supervisor" of the process. The Etheric Body then communicates with the other participants and enlists their help, as needed, to accomplish the healing. These other players include the Physical Body, the Brain, the other layers of the Aura, and the Chakra System. Each of these have special functions in the healing process and the appropriate one must be called upon by the

Etheric Body to aid in the process. The Chakra System is a major player because of its unique role as the distribution system for energy flow throughout the body.

However, even though the Etheric Body may know what is wrong and what needs healing, it won't act unless told to do so. The key to Bio-Etheric Healing is that we ourselves, or a healer, must give the Etheric Body directions as to what to do and it will do it.

When the Etheric Body is asked to heal something, it does the best it is able to do with the information it has. The more information provided to the Etheric Body, and the greater the accuracy of the information, the better it can accomplish its healing role.

This section outlines the role in Bio-Etheric Healing played by the Aura, with its critical first layer, the Etheric Layer or Etheric Body. Other important participants which will be covered are the Physical Body, the Brain, and the Chakra System. To understand Bio-Etheric Healing and how it works, it is important to first understand some basic information about all these major participants and their roles.

THE AURA AND ITS ROLE IN BIO-ETHERIC HEALING

On this planet, Earth, every form has an Aura, all people, plants, inert objects, minerals, et cetera. All have this radiating field of energy we call an Aura which surrounds all things in our physical environment and surrounds our bodies as well. Most of us can't see this field of energy. Some "sensitives" and clairvoyants can see this Aura and may understand what the different colors and forms in this shimmering mass of light might mean. For most people, this ability is below their level of awareness. Some children are born with this ability but since this is not shared or understood, adults frown on it and children lose this ability at an early age. Prehistoric man may have had the ability to see or sense the Aura as evidenced in cave paintings of figures with halos or radiating lines coming from the body. This radiation of vital energy from all life forms has been accepted from antiquity with references to it in the writings and the art of India, Egypt, Greece, and Rome.

The Aura that surrounds us contains our personal history, including past and present Traumas, Karma, and all aspects of our health.

It surrounds us like a giant, colorful egg, extending out about sixteen inches from our bodies. It is made up of gaseous matter, all held together by a delicate web. It manifests in different shapes or hues depending on how we feel, mentally and physically.

Edgar Cayce, a well-known and respected psychic of the early twentieth century, saw Auras beginning in his early childhood and throughout his adult life. For the longest time, he thought everyone had this ability. The colors enchanted him and he tried to identify their meaning. After years of study, he realized that both the physical and emotional health played a part in the changing palette. He was saddened when seeing an Aura in shades of grey, for color meant life, and grey meant the end of life.

Kwan Yin said, "Within the Aura lies the key to our health." Before any illness or physical problem manifests itself in the body, it first appears in the Aura. This predictive characteristic of the Aura has been documented with Kirlian photography of a plant and its Aura which picked up an outline of a leaf in the plant's Aura before the leaf became fully visible in three dimensions.

In recent years, more has been learned about the Aura. There exist seven visible layers and two that are known to exist but are barely visible. It is in the first layer of the Aura, the Etheric Layer, that most of our healing work is accomplished.

As this Aura is an energy field that surrounds all things throughout the world, it is possible to connect into the energy field of another person (his Etheric Body) over distances in order to communicate healing messages. This is comparable to direct dialing in our hard-wired electrical energy communication field. Thus helping another person who needs healing can be accomplished over distances and does not require face-to-face contact.

Another aspect of the Etheric Layer of the Aura, that is, the Etheric Body, is that it is also the "over soul" that lives on after we die. After leaving the Physical Body to return to the Astral Plane, the Etheric Body may eventually connect with a new physical entity for another lifetime on earth. It brings with it knowledge of its past lives and even future lives. This Etheric Body has a personality and base of knowledge accumulated from many lifetimes.

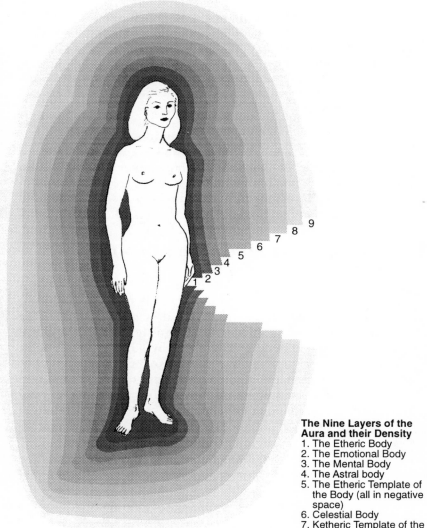

The Nine Layers of the Aura and their Density
1. The Etheric Body
2. The Emotional Body
3. The Mental Body
4. The Astral body
5. The Etheric Template of the Body (all in negative space)
6. Celestial Body
7. Ketheric Template of the Body
{ 8. Have no name -
  9. Karma Resides Here

Much of this information has been written about before (see Bibliography). However, in my work via direct communication with my own Etheric Body and that of others, I have discovered a critical new characteristic of the Etheric Body. This characteristic has laid the foundation for my development of Bio-Etheric Healing. It is that the Etheric Body is very interested in the health of the Physical Body and wants to do whatever it can to help keep it healthy or help heal it when it needs healing.

However, even though the Etheric Body can help in the healing, it usually doesn't act to help until it is asked to help, and told what to do. It actually can help in the diagnosis itself when you ask it the right questions. This interactive communication with the Etheric Body, its interest in and participation as a partner with you in achieving good health, all under your direction, is what Bio-Etheric Healing is all about.

LAYERS OF THE AURA AND THEIR ROLE IN BIO-ETHERIC HEALING

The Aura consists of nine layers which are enumerated from the one closest to the body outward, that is, the first layer is the one closest to the body. Of the nine layers, the closest seven layers are the main layers and each has its own unique function. These closest seven layers to the body are referred to by number, as well as by name. The other outer two layers which go to make up the nine do not have a name. Little is yet known about them, except it is in these outer two layers where a person's Karma resides. All together the layers of the Aura extend out about sixteen inches from the Physical Body.

First Layer — The Etheric Body

The Etheric Body, reaching out three to six inches from the body, is the first layer of the Aura. If you hold your hands at a distance from the body, and slowly bring them inward towards the body, you may feel a slight resistance at about three to six inches from the body. This is the Etheric Body. The Etheric Body interacts with the Physical Body, the Brain, and also the rest of the Aura, and can work with each of them. If you give the Etheric Body instructions, it will respond and organize the proper assistance from the other layers of the Aura, the Physical Body, and the

Brain to do the healing work needed. It promotes healing the chakras, which lie in the Etheric Body and contribute so much to general well-being. (See Chapter III.)

By working through the Etheric Body, the Physical Body can receive tremendous benefit.

- Pain due to blocked energy of a chakra or its vortices (a common culprit) may be released quickly and efficiently.
- Colds and infections may be removed easily and effectively.
- Structural repairs may be made.
- Specific chemicals may be produced.
- Injured muscles and tendons may be healed.
- Body tissue may be created.

Second Layer — The Emotional Body

The second layer of the Aura is the seat of the emotions. Working with the Etheric Body, painful emotional experiences due to circumstances in one's current lifetime may be removed from the Emotional Body. Also, tension and anxiety may be eased or eliminated by clearing the Emotional Body. Pain from emotional experiences and problems is different from physical pain, and any healing work to ease or eliminate this type of pain must involve this second layer of the Aura.

Third Layer — The Mental Body

The third layer of the Aura is the Mental Body, which is the seat of thought and intellect. All ailments which grow out of experiences in life which have created conscious thought of danger or fearful memories relate to the Mental Body. These *extreme* fears in our present life and also Traumas of past or present lives reside in this Mental Body layer. This type of extreme fear, even without conscious memory of the causal event, and even from unknown causes, creates blocked energy in the Heart Chakra, affecting the health of the person involved. It can also cause impaired functioning of the immune system. Colitis and rheumatoid arthritis are examples of common illnesses where fear is implicated. Working through the Etheric Body, a person can ask for the release of anxiety at the Mental Body level (as well as the Emotional Body level) and ask this to be done simultaneously.

Other mental problems, such as obsessive behavior patterns, can be addressed at the Mental Body level via the Etheric Body.

Some mental problems also involve an imbalance of one or more of the chakras, usually the Crown Chakra (#7) or the Third Eye Chakra (#6). Therefore, it is important to investigate whether a chakra malfunction is involved in order to know what specific approach to use.

Some mental problems require frequent repetition of Bio-Etheric Healing procedures and take much longer for improvement.

Fourth Layer — The Astral Body

The fourth layer of the Aura is referred to as the Astral Body. It is the seat of love and loving feelings. In all healing, love is a powerful force. This is true for Bio-Etheric Healing also as it is work done through the vehicle of love. The Etheric Body will not respond to request for help in healing if the request is not made with love and the total absence of any negativism. Without this atmosphere of love, the Astral Body level shuts off the healing and no progress is possible. The Astral Body level functions as a valve that makes healing possible where there is love.

Fifth Layer — The Etheric Template Body

The fifth layer of the Aura is called the Etheric Template Body. It is a template (or blueprint) which is an exact replica of everything in the Physical Body, but in the *negative* dimension. All spiritual surgery starts at this layer of the Aura. Bio-Etheric surgery actually creates "negative" space in the Etheric Body to make room for what is to be removed from the Physical Body. This surgery at the Auric level, when used with medical surgery, may accelerate healing at the physical level. Surgery at the Auric level can be used in cases where medical surgery is not possible or desirable offering the possibility of relief in such circumstances. However, this requires an extended period of time.

The Etheric Template Body used in Auric surgery needs to be used in conjunction with the seventh layer (Ketheric Template Body) which is called upon for help in the necessary follow-up repair and reconstruction of the affected area.

Sixth Layer — The Celestial Body

The Celestial Body layer of the Aura is similar to the Astral Body layer in that they both relate to love and feelings of love. However, the Celestial Body layer is concerned with love on a global basis. It is love for humanity that it involves, as well as activities that relate to the planet. Examples of this are concern with the Rain Forest, ecological systems, the well-being of animals and plants and every living thing. Generally speaking, this layer plays little or no role in Bio-Etheric Healing.

Seventh Layer — The Ketheric Template

This layer of the Aura is a template (or blueprint) providing an exact replica of the healthy Physical Body in positive space. Its primary function is to regenerate healthy cells for the body in the normal process of life. Also, it plays an informational role in healing where repair or reconstruction is needed. It provides the data to the Etheric Body as to what exactly needs to be done in the repair in order to conform to the healthy body's blueprint. This information provides the direction for the healing process.

In repairing any structural problems of the body, you ask the Etheric Body to use the Ketheric Template as a guide to define the specifications of the needed repair. In this way, the Etheric Body may ask the Physical Body to place cartilage or collagen where needed. It may remove foreign matter that is injurious to the body. It may reduce neuromas or non-malignant growths in the body and help to remove them as well.

When repair also involves a missing or a damaged cell, this layer of the Aura plays the same role in defining the specifications. This includes working with brain cells and their malfunctioning or loss.

The informational role in healing played by the Ketheric Template providing the specifications for needed repair and reconstruction was not known to me at first. This very useful knowledge was a missing piece channeled to me by Kwan Yin at a time when the specific need for it arose.

The Two Outer Layers of the Aura

The two outermost layers of the Aura have no names, but they are layers 8 and 9. They are barely visible to clairvoyants. However, they are very important in Bio-Etheric Healing, because within these two layers reside the accumulated Karma, both good and bad, of our past lives and current life.

Bad Karma often plays a determining role in certain illnesses or life situations. With Bio-Etheric Healing, it is possible to remove the detrimental effects of bad Karma in such situations. As the influence of Karma is primary over any healing, until this Karma is cleared from the two outer layers of the Aura, optimal results cannot be achieved.

Besides its role in healing, Karma affects the quality of our lives in many ways: emotional, mental, physical, as well as our social and business relationships and endeavors. It can make the difference between success and failure in these areas.

Therefore, it is always a good idea to ascertain through the Etheric Body whether bad Karma is a factor in any ailment or situation with which you are working.

THE ROLE OF THE PHYSICAL BODY IN BIO-ETHERIC HEALING

By the "Physical Body" is meant the whole organized physical or material substance of ourselves, which operates as our human form. It consumes oxygen, liquids, and foods and, in turn, produces every tissue, bones, blood cells, necessary chemicals and nutrients, and discharges its waste materials. In Bio-Etheric Healing, the Physical Body is called upon by the Etheric Body to carry out some of these same functions, specific to the healing needs requested of the Etheric Body.

For example, some of the functions the Physical Body may do under the direction of the Etheric Body would include:
- create medications for the body to use
- strengthen and relax muscles and tendons
- help the body to heal itself better and faster in most instances
- lubricate the joints
- lubricate the eyes
- produce collagen
- repair bones and tissue
- other functions mentioned under individual healings (See Chapter VIII — "Bio-Etheric Healing Applied to Specific Ailments)

THE ROLE OF THE BRAIN IN BIO-ETHERIC HEALING

Although part of the Physical Body, the Brain has such a unique function as the main electronic switchboard to receive and send signals, store information in memory, et cetera, that it plays a separate and singular role in Bio-Etheric Healing. This role relates to the particular functions which its normal operation governs. Therefore, the Brain may need to be called upon in Bio-Etheric Healing for particular healing or repair situations when a malfunction exists or a breakdown occurs. These may include:

- remaking connections for the neurons of the brain, where needed
- making new neuron connections
- helping reverse some memory loss
- helping some vision problems
- helping some problems due to dysfunction of the brain cells

THE CHAKRAS AND THEIR ROLE IN BIO-ETHERIC HEALING

The Chakra System is a major player in Bio-Etheric Healing and is involved in a large proportion of all such healing work. This is so because the Chakra System with its major chakras, lesser chakras, and their vortices, serve as the supplier and distributor of energy through the Physical Body which needs it for good health. Without the proper flow of energy in the right amount, at all times, to all the areas of the body, ill health is sure to result.

It is because of their great importance that the chakras and their role in Bio-Etheric Healing will be covered separately and more fully in the following chapter.

The Chakra System is mentioned here to complete the list of players who participate in Bio-Etheric Healing.

Chapter III

THE CHAKRAS
MAJOR PLAYERS IN THE HEALING PROCESS

> The New Medical Science will be outstandingly built upon the science of the [chakra] centers, and upon this knowledge all diagnosis and possible cure will be based.
> — Alice Bailey, *Esoteric Healing*

> What one must recognize is that the chakras are the source of power that determines the physical, mental and emotional make-up of the individual, and as such they are the key to well being... This can only be done in the light of an understanding of the chakras and their relationship to all bodies, dense and subtle.
> — David V. Tansley, *Radionics and the Subtle Anatomy of Man*

OVERVIEW

The word "chakra" comes from Sanskrit and means "wheel." Chakras are not visible to the average person, and yet they have been described by different people in different ways throughout history. They have been visible to some mystics and clairvoyants since ancient times. Barbara Ann Brennan in her book, *Hands of Light,* illustrates the chakras as swirling cones, coming out of bands that surround the body, at different junctions, both front and back. They are cone-shaped vortices, with their pointed ends closest to the body, tying into the spinal column, and the wider, open ends pointing away from the body, and interacting with the layers of the Aura. They have been described as whirling wheels or discs of color and they are centers of energy.

These discs indicate the major chakra areas of the body and they appear to be just above the body's surface. Each chakra is distinguished by the color of its rotating disc. The chakras sometimes radiate an energy that can extend as far as twenty feet away from the body.

The chakras are outside of the Physical Body and are part of the Etheric Body. They form an invisible energy system that controls the endocrine and exocrine systems of the Physical Body. The energy comes in through the Crown Chakra (at the top of the head) and is distributed throughout the body via the Chakra System.

In Bio-Etheric Healing it is important to understand some basic facts about how these chakras work, their function, and how you can learn to make them work for you to insure good health.

1. There are seven major chakras, two lesser chakras, and there are over nine hundred vortices, some very small. This system extends throughout the Etheric Body — all radiating energy. However, problems can occur in the proper functioning of this system of energy flow and distribution.

   When any such disruption occurs, it may result in discomfort, pain, generally poor health, and even contribute to the development of specific illnesses or diseases.

2. There are four potential conditions which can interfere with or disrupt the proper flow of energy in the Chakra System, that is in one or more chakra(s) and/or their vortices:
   - *Blockage* of the chakra
   - *Imbalance in activity* of the chakra
     - Underactivity
     - Overactivity
   - *Cloudiness* of the chakra
   - *Damage* to the chakra

3. These conditions can sometimes develop within a chakra or its vortices for unknown reasons, or can result from outside conditions or events which can affect the Chakra System. These outside conditions or events include factors that are physical (such as an accident), psychological, emotional, as well as factors such as foods, chemicals, toxic materials, et cetera. Another set of factors, which are technically outside factors, but we need to delineate them here for their impor-

tance in understanding Bio-Etheric Healing are illnesses, Miasms, Karma, and Traumas of past and present lives. In Chapter VIII, a fuller discussion of all these factors and their interaction with the Chakra System is given as it relates to their contribution to a particular ailment.

4. The important point to make here is that the *health of an individual, both physical and mental, depends directly upon the health and proper functioning of the Chakra System.* It is essential to keep the chakras and their vortices *unblocked, balanced, clear, and undamaged.*

DISCUSSION OF EACH CHAKRA AS RELATED TO YOUR HEALTH

Following is a discussion of each chakra, its functions, the parts of the Physical Body to which each is related, and also the specific health problems that are related to each.

Specific healing with each individual chakra is not covered in this section as many health problems relate to more than one chakra. Also with Bio-Etheric Healing the necessary healing work may involve other participants besides the chakras, such as the layers of the Aura, the Physical Body, the Brain, et cetera. Indeed, other actions, such as the need for nutritional support, as an adjunct to Bio-Etheric Healing might also be required or suggested.

Therefore, the suggestions for remedial action and healing work for specific health complaints, ailments and diseases are covered in Chapter VIII — "Bio-Etheric Healing Applied to Specific Ailments." It teaches ways to use the Etheric Body to help diagnose the problem, provide insights as to which facts are involved and what steps need to be taken to help.

ENERGY RADIATING FROM THE CHAKRA ENERGY DISTRIBUTION SYSTEM

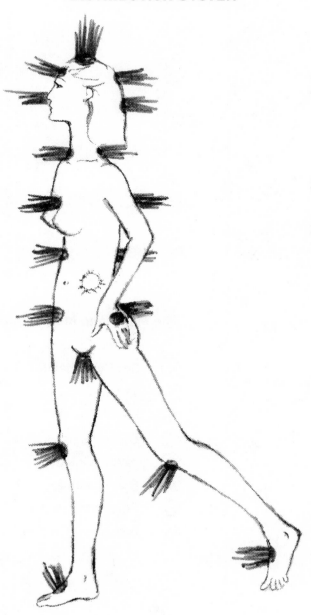

The Chakra System Used for Bio-Etheric Healing

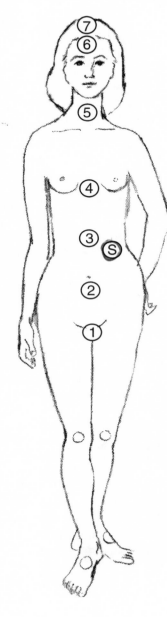

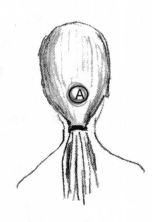

The Major and Minor Chakras

⑦   Crown Chakra

⑥   3rd Eye Chakra

⑤   Throat Chakra

④   Heart Chakra

③   Solar Plexis Chakra

②   Sacral Chakra

①   Base Chakra

Ⓢ   Spleen Chakra

Ⓐ   Alta Major Chakra

◯   Other Important Chakras

Base Chakra — #1

The Base Chakra is located at the apex of the sacrum at the base of the spinal column between the genitals and the anus. The healing color is red, and the gland it governs is the adrenal gland. Its purpose is to protect the Physical Body from harm through the adrenal gland's ability to produce adrenaline immediately when needed to energize the body to fight off any attack. A malfunction of the adrenal gland may cause allergies and so allergies are related to the health of the Base Chakra also. This chakra, in addition, affects the kidneys, spine, nerves, and the inner layers of the skin. Overstimulation of the Base Chakra is sometimes involved in mental problems. Toxins from bacterial and chemical sources can reside here in the form of Miasms along with true Miasms (predisposition for diseases).

Of the major illnesses prevalent in the world today, each illness has its own Miasm. Sometimes the Miasms are due to childhood diseases, sometimes caused by the Etheric Body of a person picking up a Miasm from being near someone who has a particular disease. If a disease is common in your area, chances are you have a Miasm for it.

Miasms can also be the result of the body's absorption of toxins, chemicals, and other compounds over a long period of time. Tansley suggests that the prevalent medical use of such compounds as alkaloids, antihistamines, hormones and antibiotics, as well as X-rays, can deepen a Miasm. I suggest that chemotherapy and radiation can also be included in this list.

As Miasms reside in the Base Chakra, they also affect the endocrine system and the adrenal gland, thus interfering with the optimal performance of these important organs. The more Miasms a person has in his Base Chakra, the more prone that person is to illnesses, and also the weaker the adrenal gland becomes. You can determine what Miasms are in your Aura by making a list of the family illnesses and the childhood illnesses you have had. This can provide you with clues to any remedial work you may need in terms of what Miasms need to be removed. (See "Miasms" under Chapter VIII — "Bio-Etheric Healing Applied to Specific Ailments.")

Some examples of Miasms are:
  • cancer
  • rheumatoid arthritis

- shingles
- scarlet fever
- diphtheria
- chickenpox
- Epstein-Barr Syndrome
- fungus infections

You can determine which of these Miasms are in your Base Chakra by using your Communications Skills, which will be described in Chapter IV.

Miasms are the predispositions (or preprogramming) for a particular disease, and they manifest themselves by causing congestion and clouding of the Base Chakra, where they reside. They interfere with the maximum functioning of the Base Chakra and are important to mankind, in that if a particular Miasm is removed from a person's Aura, the likelihood of the person getting the disease is dramatically reduced (about 70%) and could greatly alleviate the suffering from those diseases as well as lengthen the life span.
— Channeled by Kwan Yin, September 17, 1994

Sacral Chakra — #2

The Sacral Chakra is located at the base of the lumbar, mid-sacral spine. Its healing color is orange. Its related gland is the gonads. The objective of the Sacral Chakra is the continuity of the race. It affects the reproductive system and directs the sexual instinct.

The Sacral Chakra governs our sexual glands and organs, and the state of this chakra and its vortices has a direct influence on our sex lives. When this chakra is clouded or blocked, the quality and quantity of our sexual experiences are affected. The under or overdevelopment of the Sacral Chakra also has an effect on our sexuality. The underactive chakra can very well limit our enjoyment and sexuality, while an overactive chakra may cause promiscuity. An underactive chakra may also be the cause of frigidity. To have this chakra and its vortices balanced and cleared then takes on a very special significance to how one leads one's sexual life. To get the most enjoyment from our sexual experience requires that the Sacral Chakra be in a healthy state. You can ask your Etheric Body to clear, balance and heal or unblock the chakra.

Solar Plexus Chakra — #3

The Solar Plexus Chakra is located on the spine below the level of the shoulder blades, and below level of the breast bone. Its related color for healing is yellow. The gland it controls is the pancreas (stomach). The Solar Plexus Chakra is the clearing house for all energies that fall below the diaphragm. Dysfunction in the form of underactivity, blockage, or damaged chakra and vortices in this area have often been implicated in growths and cancer development. This chakra also affects the blood stream as well as the nervous system, abdominal viscera, the liver, stomach, gall bladder and digestive tract.

Overstimulation of the Solar Plexus Chakra can also lead to skin eruptions, mental problems, liver, gall bladder, stomach, and emotional problems. Damage to the coccyx can bring about damage to the Solar Plexus Chakra. Traumas from past lives, or the present life, as well as surgery, or psychological causes can result in damage to the Solar Plexus Chakra or its vortices.

In terms of cancer and Bio-Etheric Healing, Kwan Yin provided some insights:

> If one works with the Etheric Body to remove cancer from the Etheric Body, the likelihood of the cancer reappearing in the same place or elsewhere in the body after surgery would be greatly lessened. So even if one does have surgery, chemotherapy, et cetera, it would still be advisable to get the cancer out of the Aura for a better chance of survival if one chooses to continue with this life.
>
> The danger with cancer is not in the initial surgery, but in the recurrence of the problem. If that can be halted, along with work to prevent development of new malignancy, it would save many lives. And that can be done, working with the Etheric Body balancing the chakras involved, usually the Solar Plexus Chakra. Also ask the Etheric Body to remove the Miasm of cancer from the Base Chakra.
>
> — Channeled by Kwan Yin, October 16, 1994

[More specific and complete information on cancer is in Chapter VIII — "Bio-Etheric Healing Applied to Specific Ailments."]

Heart Chakra — #4

The Heart Chakra is located between the shoulder blades, on the dorsal spine, behind the heart. The color related to it in healing is grass green and the gland it controls is the thymus. All diseases of the heart, the circulatory system, and the blood, may be treated effectively via the Heart Chakra. It helps to guide the response of the adrenal gland to stress. It affects the heart, blood, vagus nerve, circulatory system, and the immune system.

The Heart Chakra and its vortices are involved in hyper-immune and auto-immune reactions. Lupus erythematosus, rheumatoid arthritis, ulcerative colitis, and myasthenia gravis are associated with a blocked or damaged Heart Chakra or vortices. An underactive Heart Chakra may cause angina pectoris and coronary heart disease. Hiatal hernia is sometimes caused by a damaged Heart Chakra. Blocked energy of the Heart Chakra may cause angina. When the Heart Chakra is overactive, it may produce heart problems and ulcers.

Throat Chakra — #5

The Throat Chakra is located at the base of the throat. Its related color in healing is a deep, clear shade of blue, and the glands it controls are the thyroid and parathyroid. It affects the vocal area, bronchial area, lungs, digestive tract, throat, the nose, the mouth, respiration, and alimentary canal. The Throat Chakra reaches up to the medulla oblongata and down to the shoulder blades. It is essential to normal growth and controls oxidative processes and calcium metabolism in digestion.

Allergies, anemia, fatigue, laryngitis, menstrual problems, sore throats, vertigo, and respiratory problems may be related to an imbalance of the Throat Chakra, as well as damage, blockage, or cloudiness in this chakra and its vortices. Asthmatic conditions can be triggered by damage to this chakra from sudden emotional shock. Blocked energy of the Throat Chakra also may cause pain and stiffness in the neck and shoulder blade areas.

Third Eye Chakra — #6

The Third Eye Chakra is located in the center of the forehead between the eyebrows. Its related color in healing is indigo, and the gland it controls is the pituitary. It is through this control of the pituitary, which is the power center of the endocrine system involving the thyroid, parathyroid, gonads, adrenals, and pancreas, that the Third Eye Chakra also influences these parts of the Physical Body. Its relationship to the pituitary is critical because this important gland has the power to initiate action when these other glands need more hormones. It can make a particular hormone as necessary, to aid a specific gland which may be having trouble producing that hormone.

The Third Eye Chakra is also involved with use of the imagination. It affects the lower brain, left eye, ears, nose, teeth, and nervous system. Malfunction of the 6th Chakra produces serious diseases of the brain and eyes, nose, ear, and nervous system. Underactivity causes sinus problems, and hay fever. One needs to determine the exact problem with the chakra and heal it accordingly to effect change in the physical condition.

Crown Chakra — #7

The Crown Chakra is located at the top of the head. Its related color in healing is violet, and it controls the pineal gland. The Crown Chakra also contains within it a facsimile of each chakra, as well as a blueprint model of the total body.

The Crown Chakra comes to the aid of any chakra that needs help, It is seen as a master control panel for the whole body and all the chakras. It also comes to the aid of the Physical Body when needed by creating necessary cells. The Crown Chakra affects the upper brain and right eye. Malfunctioning of the Crown Chakra can produce hypertension, psychological problems, some brain disease, and nervous disorders.

Two Other Important Chakras: Spleen and Alta Major

Although not included as major chakras along with the other seven, the Spleen Chakra and the Alta Major Chakra, nevertheless play an important role in our body's health. They do not have a number.

Spleen Chakra

The Spleen Chakra is located at the left side below the last rib. The gland associated with it is the spleen. The Spleen Chakra vitalizes the Physical Body via the blood stream. It manufactures white blood cells and stores iron.

Alta Major Chakra

The Alta Major Chakra is located at the top of the spine at the base of the occipital bone. The glands involved are the pineal, the pituitary, and the carotid. It is the center of energy exchange between the pineal gland, pituitary gland, and the spinal column. It affects the spinal column, carotid gland, tissue fluids, and blood pressure.

CAUSES OF CHAKRA MALFUNCTION

As noted at the beginning of this chapter, there are four potential conditions which can interfere with or disrupt the proper flow of energy in the Chakra System. These conditions are a blockage, an imbalance, cloudiness, or damage. They can occur either in a chakra or its vortices or both.

There is often little that can be done of a preventative nature to protect against some of these conditions. This is so because many of the causes of these conditions occur due to unknown reasons or from conditions or events outside of our control. The body of this book deals with keeping the Chakra System healthy where it is within our control as a preventative therapy where this is possible, or as a remedial therapy after a malfunction has occurred.

As a means of further understanding of the complicated yet vital nature to our physical health related to the health of the Chakra System, the following channeled information on the known causes of chakra malfunction is included.

Blocked Chakras may be caused by:
- Emotional factors such as anxiety, fear, shock, the stresses of daily living
- Illness that is present or imminent, or by infection
- Unresolved relationship problems
- Use of drugs, chemotherapy, or radiation
- Traumas of past or present lives, as well as Karma of past lives
- Allergic reactions to foods, chemicals, or toxins

Damaged Chakras may result from:
- The birth process itself
- Chemotherapy and radiation
- Some physical activity such as an accident, a blow, or during surgery

Cloudiness of the Chakras may be due to:
- Emotional causes (all the negative emotions are involved), such as anger, unhappiness, feeling unloved, hopeless, helpless, and powerless, et cetera.
- Rigid behavior patterns
- Miasms (in the Base Chakra only)
- Traumas of present or past lives, as well as Karma from past lives
- Allergic reactions to food
- Residues of illnesses and drugs used for treatment during one's lifetime
- Chemicals or other toxic matter in the air, or in the Aura, or in the physical body

Chakras that are unbalanced may be due to:
- The birth process and the over- or under-development of a particular chakra
- Blows to the head or body
- External life circumstances, or one's inability to adjust to changing life circumstances
- The result of gland and body changes during puberty and menopause
- Sudden changes in one's life, loss of a loved one, loss of a job, divorce, separation, emotional blows, any kind of stress
- Illness or infection
- Negative emotions, fear-anxiety, deep inner sorrow, lack of love received, Traumas of present or past lives, Karma due to past lives
- Rigidity of the thought process

— Channeled by Kwan Yin September 17, 1995

Much of Bio-Etheric Healing work has to do with working with the Chakra System to keep it healthy. This work is done by communication with the Etheric Body to ask it to do the necessary work. The same skills in communication are needed to help direct the Etheric Body in work with the other key players in this healing work (the other layers of the Aura, et cetera.)

Therefore, we need to learn about developing what we will now call our Communication Skills.

Chapter IV

DEVELOPING YOUR
COMMUNICATION SKILLS
(Talking to the Etheric Body)

Knowing the influence of the chakras on the physical and emotional health of our bodies, particularly their connection to the glands of the body, opens up the field of healing through the Etheric Body and the Aura to a greater spectrum of possibilities. These possibilities are greatly enhanced and are made more achievable by the *combination* of four discoveries during the development of Bio-Etheric Healing.

1. The breakthrough of *direct* communication with the Etheric Body.
2. The new knowledge that the Etheric Body *is actively interested* in maintaining the health of the Physical Body and is eager to help do so.
3. The new knowledge that the Etheric Body is able to provide some useful *diagnostic information,* when asked.
4. The new knowledge that the Etheric Body is able to *organize* and *direct all of the other players* (the Chakra System, the other layers of the Aura, et cetera) to do the necessary healing. However, it does not take the initiative on this, but is happy to respond to request for healing actions from us directly.

Therefore, to make the most of the great opportunities these breakthroughs present for becoming and staying healthy, there are several procedures you need to learn and master. I call these the ABC's of Bio-Etheric Healing.

These procedures are discussed fully in the pages that follow.

- Learning to communicate with the Etheric Body and make it your friend and helper.
- Using these new found "Communication Skills" to talk to the Etheric Body to help with the diagnosis.
- Using the Etheric Body to help in the healing work by asking it to do the procedures indicated.

MAKE FRIENDS WITH YOUR ETHERIC BODY — IT WILL WORK MIRACLES FOR YOU

One of life's greatest rewards is to have control over one's body and to have the power and ability to stay well. If one does become ill, to have the knowledge that may help you to heal yourself. It is sincerely hoped that what I have learned in my own personal experiences will provide you with new knowledge and tools which may help you to heal yourself and others.

I do realize that what we are talking about is working through a dimension that is not visible, yet very much there and available. It is the invisible part or dimension of yourself called the Aura, and its first layer, the Etheric Body.

Yes, it is possible! Yes, it is a reality! Yes, you can do it! For some of you it will require more faith than you now possess, but FAITH will come with success, and with knowledge, perhaps an opening to a new awareness. Most disease or sickness starts at this Etheric level and most healing starts there also. Knowing this, and trusting it, is the first step to a great adventure. It is your relationship with the unseen part of yourself that is still you.

Your Etheric Body (as I call it — my E.B., for short) wants to do anything it can to help keep you healthy. It also has the ability to listen to you, and to do your healing for you. At first, you may give your Etheric Body directions only to be amazed that it will actually do what you want it to do. Later on, if you have learned to trust your inner voice, you may get a "PING," meaning "I am here," and a voice in thought form. Your Etheric Body is many lives older than you and can communicate with a very fine vocabulary through the use of the thought process. Furthermore, since it has a voice, and does not get much chance to use it, it is delighted to have someone with whom to communicate. (I had one experience, working with the Etheric Body of a friend, over distance, whereby her Etheric Body kept talking to me and asking me questions just to keep me talking to her. Later, this same friend decided to speak to her Etheric Body herself, and was so startled when she got an answer that she stopped, and didn't try it again for some time.)

As you learn to work with your Etheric Body, and branch out to reach other people's Etheric Bodies, you will find the Etheric Body has a personality. Sometimes it is very shy and you have to be very gentle with it to get it to respond. Sometimes it is very warm and friendly and eager to have a chance to use its voice. If you reach a particular Etheric Body more than once, it will remember you, and usually greet you very warmly. It doesn't get much chance to talk to people, and really enjoys the contact, and looks forward to it. It is wonderful to make a connection with the Etheric Body of another and be greeted as an old friend! "Howdee! How are you all?" "Hi, Lady," from a two-year-old that I had worked with when he was just born!"

The Etheric Body interacts with the Physical Body as well as with the rest of the Aura. The Etheric Body is able to help with most healing work by itself but does work with the Physical Body, as well as the rest of the Aura as needed. When you ask it to do healing, it will usually engage the help of the Physical Body and other layers of the Aura. There are some situations where, if you know that other layers of the Aura are involved, it is best if you can identify them for the Etheric Body. This is especially true if you want it to use the Mental, Emotional, Etheric Template, or Ketheric Template layers of the Aura in the healing. Therefore, when you know what specific layers of the Aura are needed to help with a particular problem, it is best to tell the Etheric Body to call upon that specific layer for work as necessary.

If you tell it to do something, it never says, "I'll do it." It will say, "I'll try; I'll work on it," or something to that effect. The connection with you is something new for it, as well as it is new for you, and it hasn't had the experience to know what it can or cannot do. The Etheric Body cannot program itself or it would do so. You have to direct it.

For example, the Etheric Body works with the Chakra System to relieve pain. The Etheric Body does not feel pain itself. If you have pain, you have to tell the Etheric Body that you have pain, and where it is exactly. Say to the Etheric Body, via your thoughts, "Please break up the blocked energy causing that pain. Thank you very much." Finish by saying "Goodbye," to break the connection.

It will try the utmost to help you by working with the Chakra System to do so.

The Mental Body is involved for work with the Brain and thought processes and the release of Traumas. Also, the Mental Body is involved in obsessive behavior.

The Emotional Body is involved with psychological work. It is necessary to use the Emotional Body to get rid of simple anxiety and fear in our current life.

The 7th layer of the Aura, the Ketheric Template Layer, is used for reference when one needs to make structural changes. It has a template for everything in the Physical Body. One can ask the Etheric Body to use the information as a blueprint of a healthy body in order to know how to repair any damage, or to repair and create new cells that are damaged or missing.

Under the direction of the Etheric Body, the Physical Body can become a wondrous chemical plant. It has an ability to take the information you provide via the Etheric Body and use chemicals present in the body to produce the same medications that the body needs to help in healing. It produces these in the amounts necessary to your body's needs so that your body never receives dangerous doses of chemicals that might hurt it.

Once, having read that hyaluronic acid is used to offset the pain and stiffness of crippling arthritis, I asked my Etheric Body to produce hyaluronic acid for me, and it did. How do I know that it did? I have the ability (and will teach you also) to speak to my Etheric Body and find out what's going on. Also, the pain in my knees eased up. It seems just a few drops of that acid was necessary to do the job. My body handled that without any problem. Interestingly, months after I had asked my Etheric Body to produce hyaluronic acid, one day my knees were particularly painful and I decided to ask my Etheric Body to lubricate my knees. I had forgotten about hyaluronic acid. I asked, "What are you going to use to lubricate my knees?" My Etheric Body answered in a very low voice, "hyaluronic acid." It was incredible!

Here are only some examples of what the Etheric Body may help do for you to give you some idea of the kind of communications you can have with it.

- You can ask questions of your own Etheric Body to help you to know what needs to be healed. It will know what organs or chakras are damaged or need to be worked on. Yet it will not do the work unless you tell it to do so.

You can ask the Etheric Body of another person the same questions and receive answers also.

You can ask the Etheric Body to stop you from grinding your teeth at night.

Much pain is caused by blocked energy in the Chakra System and it may knock out or dissolve the blocked energy in minutes if you tell it to. You must give the location of the pain or chakra involved.

It may strengthen muscles and organs of the body. Just tell it what to do.

It can help knock out a cold, the flu, or other infections quickly; possibly overnight if the illness is caught early enough. Healing possibilities include infections, whether bacterial or viral.

You can ask the Etheric Body to ward off infections, bacterial or viral. You might even ask this on a daily basis which would be especially important for people in new situations, where they have not established resistance to new germs, or to people that are being exposed to new germs because of their work. This is also very important for small children going to nursery school or elementary school who are continuously contracting infections that they are exposed to.

Your Etheric Body would like to take time to get to know you, and for you to get to know it. It would love just to talk to you for awhile and, if you have the time, you might want to spend some time making friends with it. To do this, you need to develop your Communication Skills.

COMMUNICATION SKILLS

The Bio-Etheric Healing method depends on your ability to communicate on a thought level with the Etheric Body, either your own or someone else's. As we've learned, when communicating with the Etheric Body of someone else, distance does not matter. Also, it is these same Communication Skills you will sometimes need to reach and get responses from the Devic Kingdom, Nature Spirits, and Devas in charge of the lower life forms which are involved in certain ailments.

Centering — The Necessary First Step

Decide in advance which energy source (for example, the Etheric Body) you are asking to speak to, and plan exactly what you want to say. You need to physically be where you will not be disturbed. You need complete concentration. Get all extraneous thoughts out of your head and allow your body and mind to relax. Some deep breathing exercises may help to achieve this relaxation.

- Sit a short while and take deep breaths to relax. Then ask your Physical Body, via thought, to become centered; see how it feels.
- Sit for a few minutes with the tip of your tongue on the roof of your mouth.
- Hold your hands at your side, raise hands up from the elbows with the palms facing each other. Then bring hands together slowly feeling the energy field of the Aura between the hands until they touch in the center of the body. Then raise both hands up to your face with hands touching each other in a prayer position and lower hands down slowly until they separate about waist level. Repeat as necessary until you experience a feeling of complete calm. You are now centered.

Use whichever one or combination of these centering exercises that works for you before you begin to contact your Etheric Body (or any other energy source). When you are centered and ready, you will need to use your Communication Skills to ask to speak to your Etheric Body. There are four methods in our repertoire of Communication Skills.

Four Methods of Two-Way Communication

The Bio-Etheric Healing method depends on your ability to communicate on a thought level with the Etheric Body. Communicating on a thought level in other spiritual work has been referred to as Inner Speaking/Inner Listening. So as not to make things too complicated here, when I speak of communicating on a thought level in Bio-Etheric Healing, I will use these two terms interchangeably as the procedures in communicating through thought processes alone are identical. Also, for those who are aware of the concept of Inner Speaking/Inner Listening, and may have mastered it, it should make Bio-Etheric Healing work more understandable and help facilitate its use.

In Bio-Etheric Healing, we talk about a *two-way communication* between you and the Etheric Body (your own or someone else's) as well as communication with other energy sources. We may also need to communicate with the Devic Kingdom which is in charge of lower life forms, including bacteria and viruses. There are times when we may need to enlist their help in the healing process.

However, though thought processes (Inner Speaking/Inner Listening) is the only method by which we can *transmit* messages to all these other energy sources in all instances, it is not the only method that any of these sources can use in *responding* in order to make for a two-way communication with us.

There are four methods possible by which we can receive a response to the thought messages we send out, or questions we ask, that are the crux of the Bio-Etheric Healing method. These essential responses can come via:

1. A thought message in return, as in **Inner Speaking/Inner Listening.**

2. **Kinesiology,** which is a method of muscle response of the energy source being contacted, with muscle tension exhibiting strength or weakness, indicating a corresponding "yes" or "no" answer depending upon the question asked.

3. **Head motions,** which is a relatively simple method of receiving a "yes" or "no" response to any question asked of an energy source which can respond by moving your head in the appropriate way.

4. **Radiesthesia,** the art and science of dowsing with a pendulum, to receive a "yes" or "no" response to any question phrased to provide such an affirmative/ negative answer.

For the moment, let us say you choose to use the Inner Speaking/ Inner Listening method, which is the thought communication method. When you ask to speak to your Etheric Body, you may or may not get some form of acknowledgment, such as a "PING" to indicate a connection. At the beginning, you probably will not. Be patient. This may come after some degree of practice. Actually, the communication may have been completed whether there was any acknowledgment or not. Don't forget, this is new to your Etheric Body, as well as to you. If it doesn't respond, try again!

However, if you do want to have a confirmation of a definite contact, you can use either of the other methods in your Communication Skills repertoire, Radiesthesia (the Pendulum Method) or Kinesiology (the Muscle Response Method) or the Head Motion Method. If you did feel the "PING" or get the sense of a connection, you can be sure you reached the energy source you requested. Go ahead and speak to it and give it instruction as to what you want it to do using thought form, Inner Speaking/Inner Listening. If you want to ask questions and have not yet mastered Inner Speaking/Inner Listening, then use any of the other three methods to get the answers.

Using thought processes for both directions in the two-way communication is most desired as it is the most direct and convenient. However, it is the most subtle form and though one may feel comfortable with it in terms of sending out messages or asking questions, it may not be possible for everyone, or in every case, to be successful with it. Therefore, the other alternative methods are offered for those who may have difficulty in receiving a thought response or in those situations where the thought responses are not coming in or are coming in too weak to be understood. Each of these four methods are described more fully below.

Communication Via Thought Processes
(Inner Speaking/Inner Listening)

When I speak of talking with the Etheric Body and having it answer, this all takes place in thought form. We can actually hear a voice in our heads as a response (as we sometimes hear in day dreaming). This is a thought process, or thought form response, and though it is not audible in the sense that we cannot tape it, it is clearly a voice response heard in thought form. It is the voice of our Etheric Body which is responding to our thought form communication. Also, even though the voice cannot be heard outside of our own inner listening, the voice will have its own individual characteristics and will embody the "personality" of the Etheric Body which is speaking. Some voices are very low and tentative, and others are strong and clear. My Etheric Body, for example, comes through very strong, particularly now that we are such good friends. Some of your energy sources will answer in thought form with simple "yes" or "no" answers, but others may come across in thought form with whole sentences and have a rich vocabulary using words not in your everyday speech patterns. Responses may also come in visual image form or symbols and utilizing color.

Using thought processes is the most subtle form of communication and may require more practice than the other methods to feel comfortable. Yet the rewards are many. You will be able to get much more complete information, and you will be quite amazed at the intelligence of your contact.

My Etheric Body has told me that she prefers to communicate with words (mentally), but that she can do it in all ways. Most of my work has been communicating with my Etheric Body via thought processes. By now, we are old friends. Our relationship has grown. Now we are able to converse quite easily. Sometimes my Etheric Body will give me information about itself that I haven't asked for, such as, "Your skin cancer cells are now gone from your Etheric self." I was very pleased to hear that, I can assure you! It meant they would be out of my Physical Body soon, as well.

When I first started talking to my Etheric Body, she would say, "I will try," or "I don't know if I can do it, but I will try." Don't forget that this is as new to your Etheric Body as it is to you. And it doesn't quite know what it is capable of doing, yet it will try its utmost to do what is asked. It will also by itself engage other layers of the Aura, whenever that is needed, to help in its healing work.

Your Etheric Body is happy to do whatever it can to make you well. It has a mind of its own, as well, but needs to be directed. It welcomes your suggestions. It also enjoys communicating with people, even others besides yourself. When I talked to my son's Etheric Body in Texas (I'm in New York State), it said to me, "I really enjoy talking to you. It gives me a chance to use my voice, which I don't get to do every often."

Two-way communication via thought processes is accomplished via these several steps:

- Have the information you want and the questions you want to ask worked out in advance as much as possible.
- Find a quiet place and time when you will not be interrupted.
- Get into a meditative, inward mood, clearing your mind of all extraneous thoughts. Then get Centered.
- In this Centered state, contact your Etheric Body by phrasing the message in thought form, "I wish to speak to my Etheric Body."
- There may be some form of acknowledgment, but not always, so be prepared for any such clue in any form, such as a

"feeling," a "ping," or some visual effects. If no acknowledgment is received, you can quickly and easily use any of the other three methods to confirm contact, if you wish.

- In any case, assume contact and move forward to ask your first question. As above, phrase the question in your mind, in thought form, and address it to your Etheric Body.

- Await an answer. It will come to you as a mental message forming in your mind and making itself heard by you in this thought form. (It is not unlike the conversations we have while in a day dream). Although responses will usually be in this thought form method, some people have experienced responses in visual form, such as symbols or color. For example, a stop sign or a red light to mean "no" and a green light to mean "yes." So be prepared!

- Then, wait a short while for the Etheric Body to get ready before continuing to ask each question you have prepared. You may find it necessary to follow up each response further to explore your problem or ailment and what needs to be done to help with it.

Kinesiology (The Use of Muscle Tension Response)

Kinesiology is used by some chiropractors, psychologists, dentists, and medical doctors to help them diagnose patients on a nonverbal level. It is a useful diagnostic tool and one that almost anyone can learn to use and to apply in self-help work as well. This technique usually involves the participation of a practitioner and the client. However, there are also techniques where you can do Kinesiology by yourself, for yourself. I'll teach you techniques using your fingers so that you may do testing for yourself, as well as for other people.

Very often I use Kinesiology myself as it is simple and doesn't require the stillness of Inner Listening. I also feel comfortable with this method. No matter when or where I am, I have my fingers available and most people are unaware of what I'm doing.

Kinesiology depends on muscle response, whether a muscle tests weak or strong. Yet it is *not* a measure of one's strength or one's will. Rather, it is a response of the energy source being contacted, reflected in muscle tension, depending on the question asked.

Be careful to avoid influencing the answer because your mind is not neutral or because of any tension in your body due to not being properly relaxed before starting.

As mentioned before, when you try to work with yourself, or someone else, you must get as much information as you can before-hand about the problem. Is it physical, psychological, or spiritual? The more questions you ask, the more information you have, the better prepared you are to figure out what to do, and what to say in order to help elicit the most useful responses for your guidance of the Etheric Body's work.

Steps In Doing Kinesiology

- First of all, plan your question so that a "yes" or "no" answer will be meaningful to you.
- A "yes" answer will be a response of strength; a "no" answer will be a response of weakness.
- An indefinite response means that the question is either worded so that a "yes" or "no" answer is inappropriate, or the energy doesn't know the answer, so try to figure this out by asking a question as to what the energy means. Such as, "Do you mean you don't know?" or, "Would you rather I didn't ask this question?"

In trying to ascertain a time frame in the past when something happened, you might say, "Would this experience have happened when I was between the ages of 1-10 or 10-20?" et cetera, narrowing it down to smaller segments to arrive at the correct time frame.

There are two alternative ways of using your hands to do Kinesiology.

Technique 1 — Description

- [If you are right-handed] Put your left hand on a flat or solid surface or on your lap with the knuckles raised. Then take the index finger from that left hand and loosely place it on top of the middle finger, keeping it in a somewhat bent position, so that the tip of the index finger sits about the center of the nail of the middle finger (this is approximate). There should be a complete lack of tension. The finger should be loose; the whole hand should be loose.
- With your left hand completely loose, ask your question. This can be done via the thought form of Inner Speaking, or it can be said out loud.

- After the question is asked, use your right thumb and index finger to try to raise the left index finger, by *gently* tugging the raised first joint of that finger. Do not try too hard, as it is not a test of strength. Do not try to pry that finger up by pulling it up by the very tip of the index finger, but rather tug gently at the first joint. The left index finger will respond for the energy source you have contacted, by releasing or contracting that finger's muscle tension to indicate the appropriate "yes" or "no" answer. If the index finger holds firm in its position, the answer is "yes." If the index finger separates easily from the middle finger, the answer is "no."
- The same procedure is followed for any additional questions.

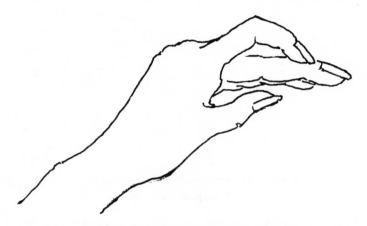

COMMUNICATION VIA KINESIOLOGY
TECHNIQUE 1

Technique 2 — Description

- [If you are right-handed] Hold the index finger and thumb of your left hand so that they touch at the tips, forming an oval.
- Take right hand and put its index finger and thumb to touch at their tips, with their tips touching just inside of the oval made by the left hand. These two touching fingers of both hands form what resembles two links of a chain.
- At this point, hold the fingers of the left hand in a very relaxed mode, touching loosely with no tension or strain. Ask your question.

- After the question is asked, keep the fingers of the right hand touching tightly, maintaining their oval link. Then try to pull the right hand out from inside the left hand "link" to see if the fingers of the left hand separate easily from their relaxed position. Do not pull too hard or try to force the fingers of the left hand to separate, as this is not a test of strength. It is only muscle tension caused by your question that is being used to indicate a response.
- If the fingers of the left hand separate easily, the answer is "No" (weakness). If the fingers do not separate easily, the answer is "Yes" (strength).

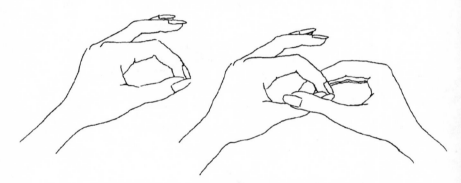

COMMUNICATION VIA KINESIOLOGY
TECHNIQUE 2

As a start, you may want to practice by asking your Etheric Body some questions. See what happens. Play with it awhile; get the feel of it; see if you can discern the difference between a "yes" or a "no." You might try asking about whether salt or sugar is good for you, and see what answer you receive.

For further ways of using Kinesiology, you can read the book by Dr. John Diamond, *Your Body Doesn't Lie.*

Head Motions

Recently my Etheric Body taught me an even simpler way of "yes" and "no" communication. I was properly centered and was starting to communicate via Kinesiology using my usual finger tension technique (Technique 1). Surprisingly, I began feeling something new and different and, in trying to understand what was happening, I found that my head was moving slightly up and down as if for a "yes" answer.

Testing this situation further, I asked my Etheric Body if this was meant to be a new way of communicating and again my head moved in a definite "yes" up and down response. I then asked if my Etheric Body wanted to use this new method to the exclusion of the other methods and I felt my head move slightly from side to side with the classic "no" response. This was clearly to be an additional method of communication.

As I have mastered the ability to relax completely and get properly centered, my Etheric Body seems to welcome this simple new method. I would recommend it to anyone who may experience difficulty mastering the more complex Kinesiology or Radiesthesia. However, as with all four methods, one has to be completely relaxed so that your own feelings or tensions do not take over the answer.

Radiesthesia (Dowsing With a Pendulum)

In using Radiesthesia to communicate with the Etheric Body by receiving answers to your questions, you must phrase the questions to allow for a "yes" or "no" response. You will, of course, be using thought processes to transmit the question or request for information. Radiesthesia is a means of receiving a response, that is, providing a method for the Etheric Body to answer you.

Radiesthesia, the art and science of dowsing with a pendulum, has been used for over 5,000 years. The ancient Chinese used the pendulum for dousing to locate the right place to put their houses. The Egyptians used it to receive answers to their mysteries. Radiesthesia is still used today in Europe to douse for water sources and to solve crimes and find missing persons. In France it is used to check on the maturity of wine.

In the Puerto Rican community, when they have baby showers, they use a dowsing method to determine the sex of the unborn child. They thread a needle and make a knot at the other end. Holding the thread by the knot, they dangle the threaded needle over the wrist pulse of the pregnant woman and hold it until it is absolutely still. Then they watch the needle start to move. If the needle goes around in a circle, it will be a girl. If the needle moves in a straight line, it will be a boy.

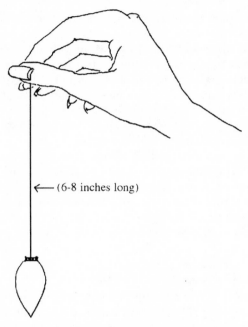

← (6-8 inches long)

Specifically, the way the Radiesthesia method is used to receive responses is by the use of a pendulum whose movements reveal an affirmative or a negative answer to your questions. The pendulum can be as simple as a weight on a string. The ideal length would be six to eight inches. A carpenter's plumb line makes a good pendulum, or something shaped like a top hanging on a string. It is good to have a point at the bottom. It can be made of wood, plastic, steel, crystal, or even ivory. It is advisable to choose one that is well balanced. Find one you like that feels comfortable to you.

You must start with the pendulum held between your fingers with the string and the weight hanging straight down and at a full rest position in mid air.

Then you need to establish with your Etheric Body what motion of the pendulum represents a "yes" answer and which motion represents a "no" answer. This is done by asking the Etheric Body to respond by giving you a "yes" response. For me, a clockwise motion was "yes," counterclockwise was "no." Check your pendulum for its answer to you.

Some Comments About All Four Methods of Communication

All four of these methods work through the Etheric Network, and can help you contact the Etheric Body or any other energy source you want to check out. When properly used, these methods make it possible to have a two-way conversation with your Etheric Body (and that of others who may be in the same room or even at a great distance). In this communication, the Etheric Body can respond to your questions and thus help provide insights to what ails you.

You may have to ask a lot of questions in order to zero in on the actual problem, sometimes via the process of elimination.

In the same way, by asking questions of the Etheric Body, you may get responses that can direct you as to what you need to tell the Etheric Body to do for you in order to help in the healing. For example, you can ask if the problem involves one or more of the chakras. Subsequent questions can identify the specific problem with the chakra(s) involved so that you may then ask the Etheric Body to carry out the necessary remedial action.

Another example is the frequently occurring situation of simple pain. As most pain is caused by blocked energy, it is important to verify if this is the case. If so, the Etheric Body may be called upon to release the blocked energy in the affected area, thereby offering relief. Other type of pain beside that related to the simple problem of blocked energy may require more investigation.

Thus, in a very real way, the right questions can help you diagnose the problem, tell you if it's physical, mental, emotional, or a combination of factors. They can direct you to which layer or layers of the Aura you need for help with the problem. You just have to be very clear with your questions so that the answers you get are meaningful.

Now you are ready to begin the diagnostic questions. You must carefully design your questions to get a "yes" or "no" answer. Keep in mind the limitation that the Etheric Body cannot discern time periods in the present or future. It can handle questions of time referring to the past. Keep asking questions to narrow it down to alternative blocks of time. For example, if you want to get information about your early life experiences going back in time, ask "Would this experience have occurred more than five years ago?"... "ten years ago?", et cetera.

Some Cautions In Communication With The Etheric Body

Though one can establish a good relationship with their Etheric Body, there are some special limitations and cautions which I have discovered in my experience which are important to mention. A lack of awareness of these or failure to appreciate their importance can cause misinterpretation, confusion, and frustration in this delicate communication process.

1. The Etheric Body does not like to be asked the same question more than once in a short space of time, either for confirmation or for any other reason on your part.

2. It is important not to overload the Etheric Body with too many things to do at one time. If you do, it will not all get remembered or done. Also relevant here is the fact that the results of the healing work may leave the Physical Body utterly exhausted, depleting its energy. For both reasons, it is best to plan your requests, asking for only one or two procedures at a time and spacing them accordingly. In fact, you can ask the Etheric Body, itself, if it is ready for the next procedure you wish to request.

3. In work dealing with the chakras, again, use caution and discretion not to try to do too much at one time. In this case, the Etheric Body may be able to do the work, but the Physical Body may fall under too much stress and become very tired. In all cases, then, moderation is the best approach.

4. The Etheric Body will not respond to any requests for information it may consider too frivolous or questionable from a moral or ethical standpoint. It will not answer questions asked strictly for personal gain.

5. The Etheric Body can respond to questions regarding time frames for periods in the past, if they are narrowed down for it in terms of alternatives. However, it seems to have difficulty in discerning shorter time periods for the present and the future.

6. The Etheric Body will not honor requests for help unless the requests are made with an attitude and presence of love and the total absence of negativism. It will simply not respond.

7. Finally, you should be forewarned that in the communication with your own Etheric Body (or that of others), you can expect a great variety in the method and content of the

responses. Expect some interesting surprises, but try not to be surprised and try to work with whatever you get.

From the workshops I've conducted and the individuals I've taught to do this work, there seemed to be no pattern for the nature of the responses. While I felt a "PING" that indicated a connection, others felt a "sense" of a connection, while others felt nothing specific.

One woman was able to actually see what she felt was her Etheric Body, describing it as a pink shell that bobbed up from behind to half cover her head every time she talked to it.

Some people were given visual images rather than a verbal response. One man described a scene where a little man similar to an elf, dressed in green, was trying to show him what needed to be done to his friend's back for healing, by pointing a huge icicle to a spot that needed attention (apparently indicating an application of a cold compress).

One other person, in response to a question that said, "Do you have a message for my friend?", received a visual symbol of a bag of sugar with a huge red "X" across it. (She should keep away from sugar.)

We know that the Aura does change color, and the colors are reflective of the emotions a person is feeling. However, all of my students agreed that despite the variations in the types of responses, that the important thing regarding this communication work was practice. The more practice they had, the more they were able to communicate well with their own Etheric Body and that of others.

Once you have mastered your Communication Skills, be they any one of the forms described, Inner Speaking/Inner Listening, Kinesiology, Head Motions or Radiesthesia (or combinations of them), you will be ready to work closely with your Etheric Body to help in the healing work.

The following chapter tells you how to use Bio-Etheric Healing to help yourself and others. You may follow the suggestion given there to develop your own knowledge and healing skills and gain new insights with your growing experience. Also, for your guidance with specific ailments or ailments which may arise and be a challenge, you can refer to Chapter VIII — "Bio-Etheric Healing Applied to Specific Ailments."

Chapter V

USING BIO-ETHERIC HEALING
TO HELP YOURSELF AND OTHERS

HEALING YOURSELF
WITH YOUR OWN ENERGY FIELD

As we have seen, within the energy field that surrounds you (and everything and everyone on this planet), this field we call the Aura, you have a willing helper in your quest for good health. What is more wonderful, and truly miraculous, is that this willing helper, your Etheric Body, has the capability for doing effective healing work for you under your direction.

Using the Communication Skills you just learned in the previous chapter, you can have two-way conversations with your Etheric Body discussing your health complaint so that it can be of maximum help in the situation. It has excellent diagnostic abilities if you provide it full and relevant information and then ask it the right questions.

It is capable of telling you what is making you ill, whether a malfunction of the Chakra System is involved, whether a particular chakra needs to be healed, or if the gland related to the particular chakra needs attention and what needs to be done for it.

The Etheric Body can tell you, for any ailment, if any organs or glands are affected and which ones. It will answer questions regarding Miasms in your Base Chakra and any growths that appear on the Solar Plexus level or any place else in your Aura or Physical Body. It can identify where the blocked energy is that is causing pain in the body, and many other problems and situations. Just Ask!

Your healer is always there for you, day or night, at home or riding in a bus, it is there for you. Sounds like a love song, and it is. It is the love of your Etheric Body.

In this context, then, you can begin to understand and believe that illness, both mental and physical, can start, or be the result of problems first manifested at the Etheric level of your energy field. You can also understand, then, that much healing can go on at the Etheric level, outside your Physical Body, yet it directly affects your physical being. The Aura has a blueprint of everything that is in your Physical Body, and the Etheric Body has the intelligence to follow your directions to heal itself and the rest of the Aura as well as the Physical Body.

Kwan Yin says that 99.9% of ill health begins at the Etheric level and can be healed from that level.

The chapters that follow will reveal the step-by-step procedures to help you manage to achieve better health, by utilizing this knowledge. It is an incredible self-help system by which you can help yourself without drugs, sometimes quickly, sometimes slowly, depending on the problem, and even help with problems where no known healing possibilities exist.

The Etheric Body can, and will, orchestrate the healing through its own layer, as well as the other layers of the Aura AS LONG AS YOU TELL IT WHAT TO DO! It also can, and does, work with the Physical Body and Brain directly. True, you can't help every-thing this way, but what you can help seems like a miracle! Tansley in *Radionics and the Subtle Anatomy of Man,* alludes to this capabil-ity, referring to the concept of the Etheric Body as a tool of life which shapes and sustains the physical form.

Keeping the Chakras Healthy

A good place to start in working to achieve good health is to work with the Chakra System. This is so because the chakras are involved with the proper flow and distribution of energy through-out the Aura and the Physical Body. The chakras also control the endocrine and exocrine (glandular) systems of the Physical Body. As a result, the Chakra System plays a major rule in maintaining good health and is very often involved in some way when things are not right.

This chapter will tell you how to keep the Chakra System healthy as a very worthwhile precautionary step — a kind of good-health insurance policy.

In Chapter VIII — "Bio-Etheric Healing Applied to Specific Ailments," mention is made if the Chakra System is involved in a particular ailment. It tells which specific chakra or chakras may be implicated and what to do to heal them.

For this same purpose, you can also ask your Etheric Body itself to tell you what is wrong using your Communication Skills to get an answer (see chapter on Communication Skills). Once you know which chakra is involved, ask your Etheric Body to tell you if the chakra or its vortices are not in balance (overactive or underactive), blocked, damaged, or cloudy. Your Etheric Body may know what is wrong, but will not do anything about it until you give it instructions. You will need to contact your Etheric Body and give directions to either correct the imbalance of the chakra, or remove the blockage of the chakra, or clear the cloudiness. IT WILL DO SO! If the chakra is damaged, ask the Etheric Body to heal it where possible. For very serious illnesses, this approach may not be all that the body needs, but it will definitely improve the state of health. Nothing said here is meant to preclude working under the supervision of your medical professional or with other therapies with which you are comfortable. Bio-Etheric Healing can work well as an adjunct.

There is agreement by both David V. Tansley *(Radionics and the Subtle Anatomy of Man)* and Dr. W. Brough Joy *(Joy's Way)*, that the chakras represent a focal point where energy is received and transmitted throughout the body. This knowledge underlines the importance of keeping the chakras healthy.

Keep in mind that in working with the Chakra System, what you want to achieve is to have a system of well-balanced, well-functioning chakras, no blocked energy, and no overactivity or underactivity. You can tell your Etheric Body what you need to have done to heal the chakras and it will provide the healing.

Chakras can be affected by traumatic accidents, and especially by sudden, dramatic emotional shocks. Continuous fear or anxiety creates a wear-and-tear effect which can block the energy of the chakras or their vortices. Chakras are frequently blocked at exit or entrance points to the Aura. Blockages can also be caused by Miasms or Toxins, but only in the Base Chakra.

Some other examples of how chakras relate to the Physical Body
are:

- A damaged chakra or its vortices may be involved in hiatal
  hernia.
- Heart Chakra disorders may relate to angina pectoris and
  coronary heart disease.
- Damage to the coccyx may damage the Solar Plexus Chakra.
- A blocked or cloudy Heart Chakra may be implicated in
  angina.
- Surgery can damage the chakras, depending on where on the
  body the surgery was done.
- An overactive Crown Chakra or Third Eye Chakra may be
  involved in mental problems.

Maintaining the chakras' health translates to maximizing your
own health. As noted earlier, a healthy state for the Chakra System
is one where all chakras and their vortices are:

- Clear (of cloudiness)
- Balanced (in terms of underactivity and overactivity)
- Unblocked (free of any blockage of energy)
- Undamaged (not torn or disfigured)

Kwan Yin Exercise For Health of the Chakra System

A very useful and simple exercise to help in the maintenance of
the Chakra System, at least to clear and balance the chakras and to
energize the Physical Body has been channeled to me by Kwan Yin
as follows (see illustration on page 65):

It is very simple. The suggested time to be spent on each
chakra is one or two minutes. However, if you need to go at a
slower pace at the beginning, please do so.

Also, if you can't hold your left hand six inches away from
the top of the head for the whole exercise, then place your left
hand on top of your head, when necessary.

TO START — STAND UP (If that is a problem, you can
do this exercise sitting down.)

1. Raise both arms above the head, way up high! Reach as
   high as you can. Hold it for a count (you decide), then

bring both hands down to the Crown Chakra. Leave
your left hand six inches away from the top of the head,
and bring the right hand down to a place three inches in
front of the Third-Eye Chakra — your forehead.
Hold...

2. Keeping your left hand above (or on) your Crown
   Chakra, bring your right hand down to the Throat
   Chakra, keeping it three inches away from the body.
   Hold...

3. Leaving your left hand at the Crown Chakra level, bring
   your right hand down to stop three inches in front of the
   body at the level of the Heart Chakra. Hold...

4. Leaving your left hand at the Crown Chakra level, bring
   your right hand to rest three inches in front of the Solar
   Plexus Chakra. Hold...

5. Leaving your left hand still at the Crown Chakra level,
   bring your right hand to three inches in front of the
   Sacral Chakra. Hold...

6. Bring both hands to the Base Chakra and keep them
   about three inches from the Physical Body. Hold...

7. Bring both hands to both knees, hold, then bring both
   hands down to both feet. Hold...

8. Then touch the floor with both hands.

9. Bring both hands way up above the head and feel the
   energy being activated.

— Channeled by Kwan Yin, May 15, 1995

The above is a good general exercise for strengthening the seven
major chakras. However, it is useful to add two other chakras to
this exercise when needed.

For example, at times of stress, headaches, neck pain, and infection, include the Alta Major Chakra which is at the point between
the Third-Eye Chakra and the Throat Chakra, at nose level.

Similarly, when the Spleen Chakra needs attention, such as at
times of infection, chemotherapy or radiation treatments, it should
be included. It is located on the left side of the body, just below the
rib cage.

KWAN YIN EXERCISE FOR HEALTH OF CHAKRA SYSTEM

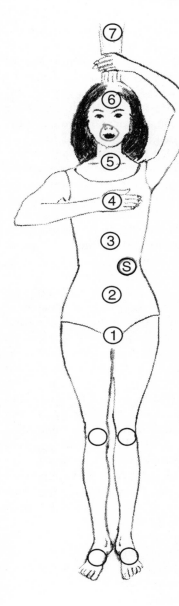

Kwan Yin Chakra Exercises

⑦   Crown Chakra

⑥   3rd Eye Chakra

⑤   Throat Chakra

④   Heart Chakra

③   Solar Plexis Chakra

②   Sacral Chakra

①   Base Chakra

Ⓢ   Spleen Chakra

◯   Knees & Feet Chakras

Diagnosing Problems

All healing work needs to start with a good diagnosis of the problem. Of course, it is best to seek the diagnosis of your medical professional when the need arises. Using your Communication Skills to work with your Etheric Body, asking further questions regarding your complaint or illness may provide a very useful enrichment of the diagnosis. This information would allow for further Bio-Etheric Healing work as an adjunct to medical treatment and help speed the healing and make it more complete.

As each individual health complaint has its unique characteristics, sometimes varying from person to person, there can be no standard procedure which can apply for everyone to follow in how to arrive at a diagnosis. This is, of course, when the problem is not a simple or obvious one such as an ingrown toenail, a headache, et cetera.

This is particularly true in communicating with the Etheric Body to explore the complaint and reach a diagnosis through the necessary method of question and answer communication. Here, too, with the simple or obvious ailments, it would be easier to know where to start and where to probe further using the background information on Bio-Etheric Healing provided thus far. One could also ask to see if any chakra is involved, which one (or ones), and what is the trouble with it. Knowledge of which gland any specific implicated chakra governs may lead to other avenues for questioning to arrive at a fuller diagnosis and allow for greater insights for the healing work required.

However, even though no complete, standardized form or list of questions, in their correct sequence, is possible to assure a good and complete diagnosis, it is useful to list suggestions for basic questions which need to be included in this search. This list of suggested questions is only meant as a checklist to include among others indicated by any starting diagnosis you may have. Also, they only represent questions that initiate an avenue of inquiry and they each might require appropriate follow-up questions, based on their response, to explore the possibilities further.

Checklist of Basic Questions As a Starting Point
   1. Is this illness related to blocked energy?
   2. Is this illness related to a chakra problem?
   3. Is this illness related to a glandular problem?

4. Is this illness related to anxiety/fears or psychological problems?
5. Is this illness due to an infection?
6. Is this illness related to an immune system malfunction?
7. Is this illness related to present life Traumas?
8. Is this illness related to past life Traumas?
9. Is this illness related to Karma?
10. Is there a reason to hold on to this illness?

Prepared with this information, and using your own ingenuity as you gain personal experience in the magic of talking to your Etheric Body, you will soon master the concept and procedures of healing yourself with your own energy field. To help in learning the many applications of Bio-Etheric Healing, step-by-step procedures for specific ailments are provided in a following chapter.

If you have not yet mastered communication with the Etheric Body well enough for the diagnostic aspects of this work, you can simply follow the procedures provided for the healing work on a specific ailment and communicate them to the Etheric Body by quietly telling it what to do. This will work for you, even if you haven't fully developed a conviction or faith in the method. It is only necessary to do this work with an attitude of love and the complete absence of negativism. If this rule is followed, you need not worry, because even if your instructions to your Etheric Body are wrong, it will not take any action that would be harmful. If your instructions are wrong, incomplete, or unclear, it will probably not follow through on them.

HEALING SOMEONE ELSE

The same energy field (the Aura) which surrounds us, and everything and everyone, and allows us to have a two-way communication with our own Etheric Body, also allows us to communicate with the Etheric Body of someone else.

It is possible! It is true! I have done it! I have taught others and they have done it!

All it takes is to master the Communication Skills which I have previously described.

It works based on the same concepts and procedures except that you are now addressing your thought messages to the Etheric Body of someone else. Remember, for this two-way communication, you are able to transmit your messages out only via thought processes (in thought form). However, for receiving responses, you have three other choices beside thought form communication, namely Kinesiology, Head Motions and Radiesthesia. Use whichever you are most comfortable with.

As a reminder, the procedures for working with someone else are the same as those for working with yourself, except for two important additions, namely:

- You must first ask the person's permission to work with his Etheric Body.
- After you have worked with another person's Etheric Body, you must tell that person what you have asked his or her Etheric Body to do. This is to help the person to understand what you are doing. Make the person aware of the fact that detoxification will probably take place, with accompanying symptoms. Drinking lots of water is a great help to getting the toxins out of the body.

If you are working with the Etheric Body of a child, speak to the child's parent or guardian to tell her or him what you have told the Etheric Body of the child to do, and advise them of the possibilities of detoxification as well.

Healing Someone Physically Near You
Here are the steps to follow:

Step 1. Ask the person you wish to help for permission to work with his or her Etheric Body.

Step 2. Plan ahead what you are going to say to and ask of the other person's Etheric Body. Keep the message clear and simple.

Step 3. Find someplace where you can be alone and uninterrupted. Sit quietly, concentrate on your goal, then get completely relaxed. Get Centered.

Step 4. While in this state, say out loud, or in your mind, "I wish to speak to the Etheric Body of (name)."

Step 5. Even if you do not get any form of confirmation of a connection at first, proceed with your questions as if you did. If you do not hear a voice in your head with a response in thought form using Inner Listening, begin using either Kinesiology, Head Motions or Radiesthesia as a means of getting a response to your questions.

Step 6. Remember, be friendly and cordial. Say "hello," "please," and "thank you." If you are not sure of what the problem is, you might ask questions to help diagnose or pinpoint it. If you do know the problem, you can proceed, being sure to ask if any chakras or their vortices are involved, naming each individually.

Step 7. If you are not sure what steps are needed for the healing work, again, ask questions which will provide guidance. Once you know what needs to be done, tell the person's Etheric Body what you want to work on, what the problem is, and ask it to do the healing work you want it to do. For example, say "John Doe has a bad cold in his nose. Please get it out of his system, whether it is bacterial or viral." That is important to say. Then add, "Please remove any blocked energy that may be involved in this as well." Be as clear and concise as possible. If you have a verbal connection, you may hear John Doe's Etheric Body say, "I'll get right to it," or "I'll try." Even if you haven't heard anything, go to closure by saying, "Thank you for your help. Goodbye."

In doing healing work on someone else, through communicating with their Etheric Body, the necessary first step, again, is to have a good diagnosis. As with working on yourself, you would start with the diagnosis of that person's medical professional if that is available. You might then augment it with diagnostic questioning of that person's Etheric Body following the discussion and suggestions provided in the previous section covering healing work on yourself. A checklist of suggested questions is given there to help with areas to explore. More specific suggestions for diagnosis, as well as for healing work for specific ailments, appear later in this book. This information holds true for working on someone physically near you or someone at a distance, which is described next.

Healing Someone From A Distance

This is fascinating to me. On a reality level, I cannot believe it really works, but it does. The reason it works is because the Etheric Energy Fields (sometimes called the L-Fields) make up a web of invisible matter that encircles our globe. This web of energy is not visible to the naked eye or through any special glasses, however, the energy involved connects everything in the universe. Our individual and collective Auras are made up of this energy. As everything and everyone has an Aura, we are all connected by energy.

This energy web allows us to reach someone living 3,000 miles away, or even further, as surely as direct telephone dialing. However, this type of very long distance communication is possible only by people with experience and proficiency in communicating via thought processes (Inner Listening/Inner Speaking) and after experiencing the "Ping" of a connection. Also, with this type of experience, sometimes a certain sense of "knowing" develops whereby a proficient Bio-Etheric Healing practitioner just senses that a connection has been made and can send healing messages and direct the Etheric Body of someone far away, even without feeling a "Ping." It is also possible, when communicating at a distance, to use your Kinesiology, Head Motions or Radiesthesia in order to get answers from the Etheric Body you are working with.

My own most unique experience with such long-distance communication occurred in 1994, when I tried reaching a trucker friend of my daughter who had disintegrated discs in his spine. He was in excruciating pain and asked me to help him. In order to continue operating his business, he and his wife set out on a run with her driving while he lay in pain in the sleeping compartment of their eighteen-wheeler truck. They were somewhere between Portland, Oregon, and San Francisco, California, when I sat down to try to help. I was in Florida. I was able to reach his Etheric Body and tell it what it needed to do. I hoped this would work.

It was a wonderful feeling to receive a message left by them on my telephone answering machine the next day. It said that he was feeling so much better that he could not believe it. He was able to take over driving himself within days. I have heard from them several times since then, telling me of his continued progress and the absence of pain. (See Case History #7 in Chapter IX.)

How to do healing work from a distance:

Step 1. It is necessary for a previous phone call or letter to get permission for you to work with the person's Etheric Body.

Step 2. Make sure you have the person's exact name and address or a photograph of that person to be able to concentrate on it. If you know the person well, you can hold a mental picture of the person in your mind.

Step 3. Have the instructions clearly in your mind of what you want the Etheric Body or Physical Body to do, or have it written out in advance.

Step 4. Try to do this work when that person is at a particular place (for example, at home and asleep) to make sure he or she is reachable and quiet, in order to make it easier.

Step 5. Then using your Communication Skills, ask your Etheric Body to make the connection for you with the Etheric Body of the one you want to help. Be sure to tell your Etheric Body the exact name and address of the person whose Etheric Body you want to reach. Your Etheric Body will then connect you, much like a long-distance telephone operator will make a long-distance connection for you. Wait for the "Ping" of a connection (or any other type of acknowledgment) and then proceed as you would for helping someone near.

Step 6. Remember, if you are not sure exactly what steps are needed for the healing work, ask the kind of questions which will provide you with helpful diagnostic information for guidance. Then, when you know what is needed to be done to help in the healing work, tell the person's Etheric Body what you want it to do.

Step 7. Finish the conversation with your long distance contact as if you were close by. Make sure to say, "Thank you for your help and efforts," and "Goodbye for now" to disconnect. You might then get in touch with your own Etheric Body and thank it for making the connection for you.

It is so exciting to get a far-away connection and it is fun to hear the first response by way of Inner Listening.

If it is the first time you contact somebody else's Etheric Body (either close or at a distance), you might hear, "Who are you?" "What do you want?" You should be prepared to introduce yourself, tell them who you are, why you are contacting them, and what you want them to do. Each voice will have its own personality and its own individual quality. When talking to the Etheric Body of my son in Dallas, it had a deep Southern drawl, and it would always say something like, "Howdy, Partner." After conversing several times, I became more personal. I asked how it felt about me contacting it. The answer was, "I'm happy you call me. I can use my voice; nobody else ever talks to me." I was delighted with this response. I felt I had made a great discovery. The Etheric Body enjoyed conversing. I already knew my own Etheric Body enjoyed our conversations, and I was finding out with my work with others that this was the universal situation encountered. With the Etheric Body, we are working with an energy force which wants to help and enjoys the experience.

Working With Infants and Children

It is not only possible, but often very useful to do Bio-Etheric Healing work with infants and children. It is useful, for example, with infants especially, who may have pain somewhere, but cannot speak to tell the parent where that pain is. In such cases, the parent often doesn't know what to do. Under these circumstances, even a medical professional may not know what to do.

The procedures for Bio-Etheric Healing work with infants and children are essentially the same as for adults. They each have an Etheric Body, as we all do, and it is possible to speak to their Etheric Body, using our same Communication Skills. In this way we can work with their Etheric Body to confirm a diagnosis and what may be needed to help in the healing. Bio-Etheric Healing may then be a useful adjunct to the work of a pediatrician in speeding recovery.

Step 1.   Get the permission of a parent or grandparent (or that of any other adult responsible for the child) to work with the child's Etheric Body.

Step 2.   If the child has seen a medical doctor and you have his diagnosis, use that information as the basis for informing the child's Etheric Body of the nature of the problem and what needs to be done. Plan ahead what you want to say.

Step 3.   Get yourself ready for the contact. Find someplace where you can be alone and not interrupted. Sit quietly, concentrate on your goal, get completely relaxed. Get yourself Centered.

Step 4. Ask to speak to the child's Etheric Body, remembering to be friendly and cordial.

Step 5. If it is not clear as to what the problem is, you can use your Communication Skills to ask the child's Etheric Body for help with the diagnosis. If you have mastered Inner Speaking/Inner Listening, you can ask your questions for a diagnosis directly and listen for an answer. If not, you may need to use Kinesiology, Head Motions or Radiesthesia to get the proper response. Ask questions about the possibilities, being sure to phrase them to require a "yes" or "no" answer.

Step 6. When you determine what healing work needs to be done, tell the child's Etheric Body specifically what the problem is and what you want it to do to help in the healing.

Step 7. After this, be sure to close your contact by being polite and cordial. Thank the child's Etheric Body for its help before saying goodbye.

Here are some of the kinds of common complaints children may exhibit and a very brief description of what may be done. These are provided here only as illustrations of the kinds of things possible in work with children. They are not meant to be complete. However, for complete directions for these same illustrations and others, see Chapter VIII — "Bio-Etheric Healing Applied to Specific Ailments," and look under the heading, Childhood Diseases.

With a simple cold or ear infection you can go ahead and ask its Etheric Body to kill the bacteria or virus causing the cold or infection.

- For colic, ask the child's Etheric Body to heal its digestive system. Also ask for the release of blocked energy causing the pain in the digestive system. You may have to repeat this again and again if the child is still uncomfortable.
- For teething discomfort, ask the Etheric Body for release of blocked energy affecting the mouth. Ask the Physical Body to make the teething painless by releasing endorphins that occur naturally in the body.

- For pain, tell the child's Etheric Body to release blocked energy causing the pain, being sure to specify exactly where the pain is.
- For chickenpox, first ask the Etheric Body to destroy the virus and get it out of the body. Then ask it to dry up the pustules and work to prevent new eruptions on the skin.
- For children under three years old, it may be useful to clear the Astral, Mental, and Physical Bodies when the child seems irritable. This is to clear matter that may have come from the Astral Body of the mother during the birth process.
- Some babies have their chakras damaged or blocked during the birth process. Ask the child's or infant's Etheric Body about that and ask for repair as needed.

Other Energy Sources You Might Work With

We have been talking almost exclusively about working with the Etheric energy which comprises the first (and closest) layer of our Aura and which we call the Etheric Body. We have found out that our Etheric Body is an energy source which we can contact and ask to do healing work on our Physical body.

As this Etheric energy is indestructible, when we die and our Physical Body ceases to be, the Etheric Body passes on to the Astral Plane remaining as Etheric energy, but in spirit form. Thus, the spirit forms of the world's gifted healers of the past remain in Etheric energy form on the Astral Plane and are available to us for any needed healing work. We can contact them via the same Communication Skills we have learned.

In my workshops and classes, there has been a small proportion of people who, try as they might, were not able to contact or communicate with their Etheric Bodies. However, in all but one of these cases, these individuals were able to contact and communicate with their Soul. As the Soul is a higher spirit than the Etheric Body and enables the Etheric Body to do the healing, working directly with the Soul will be just as effective. Therefore, if you experience difficulty in contacting the Etheric Body, try to make contact with the Soul instead.

In addition, there exist other energy sources which we can contact directly, as necessary, which are available for such healing work. It is not the purview of this book to discuss or explain these other energy sources in any detail. However, some of these have been touched upon and so I will only provide a list of them to make you aware of their existence and the possibility of their help for yourself or others you may seek to help.

Some other energy sources are listed here in no particular order:

- Pan, the Devas and Nature Spirits
- the Higher Self
- the Brain
- the Physical Body
- the individual parts of the Physical Body
- your individual Healing Angels
- the God Source
- Kwan Yin (ask for her three times)
- Ignatious (ask for him three times)
- Lady Amahl (ask for her three times)
- Jesus (ask for Him three times)
- The White Healing Light. This is a spiritual healing source of a general nature, but it can be very effective in strengthening the immune system. To access this energy, one must ask specifically for The White Healing Light to come and to focus its healing power on the part of the body where needed (for example, the immune system). For this work, one must ask for a short healing (5 minutes or so) several times a week on a regular basis. Longer healings are not suggested as this will result in fatigue.
- other personalized energy sources of your own choice

When contacting an energy source, be sure to specify exactly which energy you wish to address. Problems may arise if you are not specific. For example, you may get some "interference" from a response by your Lower Self, who sometimes likes to act as a "trickster." You may also encounter some free-floating spirit that is out to have some fun at your expense. The answers to your questions may be wrong or contradictory.

To check against this possibility, and until you learn from experience to discern true contact with the energy source you have asked to address, it is wise to follow up each question with, "Is this the truth?" If it isn't, tell the energy source you have reached to go away. Wait a few seconds, then ask again for the energy source you want to contact. Confirm if you have the proper contact before moving forward.

Chapter VI

THE DEVIC KINGDOM AND
ITS ROLE IN BIO-ETHERIC HEALING

Now that you are becoming familiar with this material and, I hope, comfortable with the unseen world, let me introduce you to the Devic Kingdom of Nature Spirits, and the Devas. For some healing problems, they are the only help available. However, they normally do not get involved with humans and their problems, even though many of the plant life and other lower life forms over which they govern often are a part of the human experience. They can play an important healing role in some human ailments and diseases, but only if and when they are addressed directly and asked to help.

The Devic Kingdom has a realm which extends over all plant life on this planet, as well as the lower life forms, fungi, insects, bacteria and viruses.

The Devic Kingdom has a ruler whose name is Pan. He is often described as having two small horns on his head, a beard, a man's body, and legs and cloven hoofs like an animal. For those so privileged, he has been seen carrying a lyre and the sound of music accompanies him. There is also a set of middle level officers who are the Nature Spirits. They are like elves and they can make themselves visible at times.

Each Nature Spirit has many different types or varieties of life forms under his jurisdiction and has a group of Devas who report to him. There is one Deva who is in charge of one specific life form. For example, there is a Deva for the sunflower, one for the green pea, one for each butterfly form, et cetera.

The Devas also have a cooperative system where they help each other. When contacted, they say they want to work with humans and want humans to know about what they do. Occasionally, they can be cross and nasty and they can play tricks on humans; however, they can also be very helpful. The gardens of Findhorn[1] and Perelandra[2] were created and are a tribute to the great achievements made possible with the help of the Devas. As they can be contrary, it is necessary to cultivate their friendship in order to enlist their help in healing problems that fall under their authority.

From my own experience in communication with the Devas, I have learned that the Devas want humans to be cordial. They want humans to be friendly and chat with them. They especially want to be treated respectfully. It is important always to thank them and to say goodbye at the end of the conversation.

For example, I once contacted a Deva to check on the progress of work with a client who had previously called on the Deva for help. The Deva complained to me that when that person had given her instruction, she never stopped to chat with her or to be friendly or in any way show appreciation.

PERSONAL EXPERIENCES WITH THE DEVAS

When I had Lyme disease, a friend suggested I talk to the Deva of the deer tick. I had just read Machaelle Wright's book, *Behaving As If The God In All Life Mattered,* and decided to give it a try. It was a fascinating experience. I was able to use Inner Speaking/Inner Listening to communicate with these spirits. Some people have been able to communicate with them through Kinesiology, phrasing questions to receive "yes" or "no" answers.

I went into a quiet place, closed my eyes, and asked to speak to the Deva in charge of the deer tick. Suddenly, I was accosted by a rude voice that sounded like a young man. He said, "Who are you

---

[1] Findhorn is a spiritual community in Northern Scotland that began on a piece of uninhabitable, barren land. Though nothing could grow in this sandy, windswept area, the pioneers invoked the help of the Nature Spirits and the Devas to start their community with life centered around their gardens. The result is the famous Gardens of Findhorn where many come to view this incredibly beautiful place. As the community grew, the Findhorn Foundation was set up which supports a study center for the learning of spiritual ways. Thousands come annually to work and study there where the focus is now on people, rather than plants.

[2] Perelandra is a 20-acre farm in Virginia that was started by Machaelle Small Wright. She has also engaged the help of the Nature Spirits and the Devas in developing her farm and her gardens which she named Perelandra. She writes of this work in her book, *Behaving As If The God In All Life Mattered.*

and what do you want?" He told me that he was the Nature Spirit in charge of the deer tick Deva. When I explained to him that I wished to speak to that Deva, he agreed to get the Deva to talk to me.

Then came an angry female voice which berated me for the fact that humans were crowding out the natural habitat of the deer. This was the way they were taking revenge on humans. I was rather taken aback, but she calmed down after awhile, and I asked her if she could get the Devas to control the spread of the deer tick. I also told her that if they didn't, man-made chemical controls might be used for this and could cause more damage to other plant and small animal life. The Deva of the deer tick suggested that I talk to her about a week later because she wanted to bring this up to the Council of the Devas, and she would notify me of their decision.

I waited about 10 days, and then I called for her again. This time she answered directly herself saying, "What took you so long?" She informed me that the Council of the Devas decided to try a policy of containment. We had a cordial contact. She said that the Devas were pleased that I had called because they wanted humans to become aware of them. They were eager for more contacts with humans.

Subsequently, I called for the Deva of the deer tick again to ask if she could get the Lyme disease spirochetes out of my body, and she said she would. Every time I called her after that, she had a summary of how many spirochetes there had been in my body and how many were still there. This went on for months, until we were down to zero spirochetes in my body. I suspected she extended this process because she wanted the human contact. I always made sure to finish my conversation thanking her for her help and saying goodbye.

I also contacted the Devas for removal of a fungus on my toenail. In time the fungus decreased significantly so I knew that something was happening. My guide in this area, Ignatious, confirmed my suspicion that Devas really can do some things very quickly, but that they enjoy the human contact and wish to prolong the process.

A SIGNIFICANT DISCOVERY

One day my guide, Ignatious, channeled to me that there is a Deva in charge of the HIV-positive virus. He said that the HIV virus is not a true virus, as a true virus is air borne, and the HIV virus is not. The cell structure of the HIV virus also differs from all other viruses and is the reason why it cannot be treated by conventional means.

I felt that this was very critical information which might open up great opportunities for dealing with this horrible threat in new ways. I wanted to find out more information.

I called for the Deva of the HIV Virus using Inner Speaking/ Inner Listening. When she responded, she had a strong voice and was very happy to talk to me. I asked her if there was any way that, as the Deva of the HIV Virus, she could help lessen its threat to mankind by removing the virus from people's bodies. She said that this was possible and that she would be happy to talk to anyone who wants to contact her. She asked that if anyone contacted her to recall the HIV virus from a particular person's body, she would need the name and address of that client. She would arrange for this recall to take place, but she warned that it would take time. As for people who already had AIDS, she said she would be willing to try, but progress depended on how much damage had already been done. She also suggested that asking the Etheric Body of the person to get their immune system working properly again would be a good combination for healing, along with her work.

The Deva also said that she felt badly that so many lovely people are affected by the virus in her charge and that so many have died so young. She will help those that contact her to the best of her ability, but said she cannot do anything until she is asked. I told her she will receive many calls and she said she would talk to everyone who called her because she loves humankind.

She explained that the virus had escaped and that she lost control over it. She can only kill the virus when she recalls it and it is out of the body. I asked her about side effects, but she said she did not know, as she's never done this before. She said it will take time, however, she did not know how much time. Again, she suggested working with the Etheric Body at the same time to strengthen the immune system and to ask the Etheric Body to heal the problems caused by the virus. I thanked her and said that I shall communicate this message to the people.

At a subsequent time, I had a conversation with the HIV Deva in which I decided to use a question-and-answer format. Here are my notes covering that conversation:

Question: Will you work with anyone who asks your help?
Answer: Yes, we will, we have the ability to do so.

Question: Are there detoxification symptoms as the virus leaves
            the body?
Answer: Yes, but everyone's detoxification may be different
            depending on many factors, degree of infection, and
            the condition of the body.

Question: How do you recall the virus?
Answer: By sound that only the virus can hear.

Question: How long will the process take?
Answer: Depending on the degree of infection, from one
            week, to weeks, to months, even years.

Question: How often should the request for healing be made?
Answer: Usually more than once. Around three times a year.[3]

Question: Can one get infected again?
Answer: A person does not get immunization when the virus
            leaves.

All this information on the HIV virus from these conversations
with the Deva in charge, as well as the channeled messages from
Ignatious and Kwan Yin, have formed the basis of the suggestions
for working with HIV cases provided later in this book.

Also integrated along with this information is information
gleaned from my actual hands-on experiences gained when I conducted workshops specifically focused on Bio-Etheric Healing with
HIV-positive individuals. Also included are the experiences of the
professional healers and infected individuals who attended those
workshops.

All this information is summarized and provided as suggestions
for working with HIV-positive cases in Chapter VIII on specific
healing applications, under the heading, HIV Virus Positive.

---

[3] Kwan Yin has, at a later time, channeled to me that checking the Etheric Body
of the person involved once a month to see if the body tests negative or positive is a
good idea. Kwan Yin also felt that contacting the Deva of the HIV Virus about
once a month to check on the progress of each individual situation was appropriate.

Chapter VII

OTHER ISSUES IN
BIO-ETHERIC HEALING

DETOXIFICATION

Detoxification is a natural by-product of healing work with the Etheric Body. As all illnesses appear in the Etheric Body, their healing often creates waste and residue and other effects. These wastes, residue and toxins must be eliminated.

The detoxification process can take many forms on the Physical Body level. It can exhibit the symptoms of a cold, or it can be a rash, smelly urine, a feeling of tiredness, the need to sleep, the need for water, or other symptoms, such as "the sweats," a mild fever, muscle soreness, et cetera. Therefore, when you are engaged in Bio-Etheric Healing work, and you seem to be coming down with anything, a cough, or cold, or any other physical problem, before you try to treat that problem, ask your Etheric Body, "Is this problem caused by detoxification?" If the answer is "yes," the healing for something else is taking place.

Sometimes, during periods of stress that arise when a body tries to eliminate toxic material connected to a particular pain causing illness, severe pain reflecting the original pain of that illness will manifest itself. *Do not be afraid. It will be of short duration.* It is caused by the sudden movement of toxins out of the body.

Getting toxic matter out of your Physical Body is often the result of the healing you have asked for and is directly related to what you are trying to heal. Be aware of its existence and be happy to rid yourself of the residues of past illnesses, toxins, or medications that are clogging up your system. Do not let it upset you. Anytime you cannot figure out what is going on with your body, ask it, "Is this detoxification?" Then, with Inner Speaking/Listening, ask your body to tell you what is being detoxified. Or, take some guesses using any of the other three methods in your Communications Skills toolbox for a "yes" or "no" answer.

Do not try to treat the detoxification as an illness in itself. However, as a means to minimize the general effects of the detoxification, you may ask your Etheric Body to help. Just ask it to do that for you.

Also, you can minimize any discomfort by supporting your body nutritionally during this period of stress. A suggested program is:

- drinking lots of water
- megadoses of vitamin C (500-1,000 milligrams)
- a strong multivitamin and multimineral
- a separate tablet of zinc (30-50 milligrams)
- a stress formula tablet (vitamin B and C)
- any version of a Pep-Up Formula found in health food stores

Detoxification can affect the Etheric Body in several ways. It can sometimes cause blocked energy and even cause cloudiness in a specific chakra which is involved in the problem being healed.

Detoxification can also cause pain in the physical body due to blocked energy in the chakra. If pain is present, ask the Etheric Body to break up the blocked energy in the chakra involved.

Also, it is wise, as a precaution, when healing involves breaking up blocked energy in a chakra, to ask the Etheric Body some short time later, if that same chakra is experiencing a cloudy condition. If so, ask the Etheric Body to clear up the cloudiness in that chakra due to detoxification.

Lastly, it is important to point out that the most prevalent effect caused by detoxification is an overall feeling of fatigue and tiredness. *If this fatigue becomes overwhelming or interferes with normal activity* and you wish relief, ask the Etheric Body to get the fatigue out of your body. Although it does not always occur, it is so often the case that it is wise to expect fatigue when you are healing yourself or, when healing others, to warn them to expect it as a precaution.

NUTRITION AND BIO-ETHERIC HEALING

As you work with Bio-Etheric Healing and your body becomes stronger, the need for medications and supplements will likely change. You may no longer need the dosages of whatever vitamins and minerals you were taking. You will have much less need of some things, but may find a need to add others for a specific purpose which will become apparent to you in the process. You may still need some vitamins and medications in certain situations, but this will probably be at lower levels.

However, it is very important in working with Bio-Etheric Healing (as it is with any physical or mental healing), that you supply your body with the building blocks it needs to do the healing. The body will make its own chemicals but the ingredients for these chemicals come from the foods you eat and the vitamins and minerals you take to supplement that food. Therefore, it is imperative that you ascertain what your changing needs may be. You must learn to use your Communication Skills to do this (or find someone else who can do this for you).

A healthy body normally produces the chemicals it needs in the proper amounts. As your body becomes healthier, normal chemical production activity will take place. However, when the body is not producing the chemicals it needs, either in times of sickness or due to stress, imbalances or deficiencies occur. Any such imbalances or deficiencies can be ascertained by using your Communication Skills to ask the Etheric Body what the situation is and what may be needed to come back to balance. Once the problem or the need is identified, you will be able to tell the Etheric Body which specific ingredients or chemicals are needed and to ask it to produce what it needs. It will do so in the proper amounts. It will also resolve imbalances if asked to do so. However, for diabetics, this will not work in the case of insulin production.

For example, in my own case, I was taking thyroid supplements for many years after a partial thyroidectomy. As my general health improved over the past three years via the use of Bio-Etheric Healing, my need for thyroid supplements kept dwindling to the point where my body no longer requires this medication.

Another factor to consider is the total effect of the combination of whatever you are taking, vitamins, minerals, homeopathic or Bach Flower remedies. The total effect must be evaluated. While your body may tell you to take specific items in answer to your individual questions, how does your body respond when you put them all together? This is a critical piece of information for you. Combinations of even some things as benign as Bach Flower remedies or homeopathic remedies can be harmful if you take more than your body dictates.

You must be alert to your body's changing needs and also to what foods you are eating to provide your body with the building blocks needed to do the healing. In the case of supplements, medications, or other remedies, you must understand the total effect in combination, as well as their individual usefulness, in healing and maintaining your body's health.

The best time to take your vitamins and minerals is some time *during* the meal. If you take them *before* the meal, they may become an irritant. If you take them *after* the meal, you may not have enough digestive juices in your body left to digest the vitamins. In either case, it may cause you discomfort.

FOODS

Our digestive systems evolved slowly over thousands of years utilizing the simple natural foods available in the environment during those times. With the Industrial Revolution, in our very recent past, came great changes in the kinds of foods and how these foods were produced. Processed foods were introduced, along with a wide array of sugars and sweetener products. Additives, preservatives, flavor enhancers, and chemicals were also added. The result of all this was a great and rapid change in the *nature* of the foods available for our consumption.

However, the slow evolutionary pace of change in mankind's body chemistry and digestive system has not changed in this short time span. This situation has created a wide disparity between the nutritional needs of our body and the nature of the foods generally available in the typical supermarket food store today.

This historical perspective is key to understanding the current dilemma in maintaining a healthy body in these modern times. Basic to good health and the maintenance of good health is the acid/alkaline balance of the food we eat, and in turn, upon the specific nutritional needs of our individual bodies, down to the cellular level.

The proper acid/alkaline relationship needed for good health is a slightly more acid environment to keep the cells of the body functioning and able to reproduce themselves. In such an environment, the body's cells actually maintain themselves better, age more slowly, and the body has more pep and drive.

If one's body chemistry is too alkaline, it can affect one in many ways. You may lose energy and also not be able to fight off illness as well. You may be more prone to degenerative diseases. Arthritis and bone loss are examples of this.

Therefore, we must provide our body with the right raw materials (the foods we eat), for it to have the building materials necessary for good health and the maintenance of good health.

Always try to buy the most nutritious food for your body. Eliminate white flour products and sugars. White flour products turn to sugar in the body. Sugar is a villain because it changes the alkaline and acid balance of the body to becoming more alkaline, thus interfering with the digestive process. It hinders the absorption and utilization of nutrients essential to a healthy body. Excluding sugars means excluding honey and other forms of sugar, including fructose and corn sweeteners which are used in processed foods.

Try to buy your foods in their natural form. The less additives, the better; and the less processing, the better. It is best to minimize the use of canned and frozen foods because of their additional processing.

When buying fruits and vegetables that are not organically grown, it is advisable to soak them in a bath of water to which a small amount of bleach has been added (one-half teaspoon of Clorox to one gallon of water). Soak for about 15 minutes. Follow this with several rinses of fresh water. This should eliminate the toxins that are on the surface of the foods caused by chemical pesticides used in non-organic food production. Peeling fruits and vegetables is an alternative.

For your information and guidance, a partial list of alkaline and acid producing foods follows:

ACID PRODUCING FOODS

vinegar
fresh fruit
meat
fish
cheeses
whole grain products
green leafy vegetables
most green vegetables
carrots
lemons/limes
strawberries
blackberries

ALKALINE PRODUCING FOODS

high carbohydrate foods
starchy foods
cakes/pies/pastries
ice cream/frozen yogurt
sugar in all forms
candy
white flour products (breads, pasta)
jams/jellies
dried fruit
rice
corn
potatoes/yams
beets/beet greens
beans (kidney, lima, navy)
bananas
fresh figs
grapes
sweet cherries
oranges, grapefruit
most fruit juices
carrot juice
ripe fruit[4]
shellfish

---

[4] The riper the fruit, the more sugar it contains, hence the more alkaline it becomes.

Chapter VIII

BIO-ETHERIC HEALING APPLIED TO SPECIFIC AILMENTS
(ALPHABETICAL BY AILMENT)

The following section provides a list of health problems and offers specific suggestions of how to use the Bio-Etheric Healing method to help with each problem. Before approaching this work, please remember to take these actions in all cases:

1. Be sure to use your Communication Skills (see section on Communication Skills) to speak to the Etheric Body of the person being helped, in order to ascertain:
    a. if the situation or problem described applies in the specific case in question; that is, confirm the diagnosis.
    b. which chakra(s) and/or vortice(s) are involved and in need of healing.
    c. if Karma is related to this problem; if it is, Karma overrides the specific treatment of that illness. Karma must be removed from the Aura before the specific treatment for the illness is applied. (Read ahead under Karma.)
    d. if Traumas are involved, and need to be removed before necessary healing procedures are applied. (Read ahead under Traumas.)
2. When dealing with another person's illness or health problem, make sure you have his or her permission before proceeding.
3. As soon as possible after you have worked with someone, always tell that person what you have done and advise him or

her that detoxification may follow as part of the healing process.

4. Requests to the Etheric Body must be simple, direct, and specific to the problem or situation.

5. Sometimes, in special situations, the Soul has to be contacted or may even respond and take over the healing. This is so because the Soul is more protective of the individual and sees the situation from a total perspective. The Soul is connected to the Etheric Body and is also directly connected to the God Source. It is in a position to protect the individual from factors unknown to the person or the Etheric Body. For example, when working with Traumas of past or present lives, permission must first be asked of the Soul who will not allow the removal of any Traumas whose removal might cause worse problems in the future.

In working with the Etheric Body, one must use caution and discretion in not asking the Etheric Body to do too many things at one time. If asked to do more than it is able to deal with at one time, it may follow only the first request and ignore the rest. If you are on the Speaking /Listening level with your Etheric Body, you can actually ask it how much it can work with at one time, and also how long to wait before making the next request. If you are not at this level of communication, then it is wise to make only one request at a time and wait for some time to elapse before asking again.

In working with the chakras, again it is wise to go slow and not try to do too much at one time. In this case, the Etheric Body may be able to do the work requested, however, the process may put too much stress on the Physical Body and seriously drain its energy level. In all cases, moderation is the best approach.

Some situations respond very quickly to Bio-Etheric Healing, while others are more long term in their response. For example, breaking up blocked energy can bring relief from pain in a very short time, while restructuring for damage repair is a long-term situation. Similarly, asking the Etheric Body to break up an infection due to a virus or bacteria may bring fast results if caught at the first sign of the infection. However, if not caught early, this same infection may need repeated requests and take longer to subdue. Also, when working with certain problems as with blood cells or brain cells (as in dyslexia), making repeated requests on a regular, or even daily basis, seems to be necessary.

Finally, there is an important caution to keep in mind. In the course of the body overcoming certain diseases or illness and getting them out of the system, a natural process of detoxification may occur. (See discussion of Detoxification in Chapter VII.)

Here, then, is a list of ailments and suggestions for how Bio-Etheric Healing may help.

ADDICTION
(Channeled by Ignatious)

Healing addiction allows you to cease wanting what is not in the best interest of the body.

Smoking

Working with the mind and the body using Bio-Etheric Healing means that you ask the Etheric Body to declare a state-of-emergency in the system. Ask the Etheric Body to have the Physical Body reject the substance of addiction by whatever means necessary to make it uncomfortable and undesirable to continue to use the substance. Then ask the Etheric Body to eliminate the side-effects of withdrawal of the substance from the Physical Body. Withdrawal symptoms should be minimized as a result. Some detoxification symptoms will occur. A hypnosis tape specifically designed to help a person stop smoking would be a valuable aide to the healing process.

Drug Addiction

Tell the Etheric Body that the drug is not welcome in the Physical Body and to reject it in whatever way possible. You can ask the Etheric Body to expel the offending substance by establishing a revulsion for the drug and to eliminate the pleasurable effects obtained while using the drug. If you are working with another's body, you must have the person's consent. This method has little chance if the person is not ready to be healed.

To remove the effects of crack cocaine in the body of a newborn whose mother is a crack addict, ask the infant's Etheric Body to clear the infant's Physical Body of the drug as quickly as possible and to bring about detoxification. Also, ask the infant's Etheric

Body to remove any Traumas from its Mental Body and bring the Physical Body back to normal functioning.

Coffee

The same methods used for smoking are useful to help eliminate coffee addiction, with one exception. The process will suddenly make the person feel unwell if he or she drinks coffee thereafter.

AGORAPHOBIA

(Channeled by Kwan Yin)

This is a morbid fear of crossing or being in open spaces. Usually, the origin of this fear is unknown to the person. Traumas of past lives or present life, as well as Karma, may be implicated. Therefore, Bio-Etheric Healing can be very effective with this problem.

To work with Agoraphobia, check the Etheric Body to see if Traumas or Karma is involved. If either is implicated, please refer to listings under Anxiety/Fear or under Traumas, or under Karma, as appropriate, before proceeding.

ALLERGIES (SIMPLE)

Allergies may be due to adrenal gland malfunction which, in turn, may involve problems with the Base Chakra (#1), the Third Eye Chakra (#6), or the Throat Chakra (#5). Ask your Etheric Body which of these chakras are involved.

If the Base Chakra and/or the Third Eye Chakra or their vortices are involved, ask the Etheric Body to break up any blocked energy and to clear the implicated chakras and their vortices.

If the Throat Chakra is involved, ask the Etheric Body to balance this chakra and its vortices.

Finally, ask the Etheric Body to strengthen the immune system, the thymus gland, and the adrenal gland. It may be useful also to take an adrenal gland supplement that is available at health food stores.

In the case of *severe* allergies, these may involve fear related to Karma or Traumas (of past or current lives.) Check with your Etheric Body to see if any of these factors are involved. If so, refer to the separate headings for Karma or Traumas in this chapter and follow suggestions provided.

In addition, it may be very useful to call upon the spirit source of The White Healing Light. (See Chapter V — "Other Energy Sources You Might Work With.")

During this entire healing period, be particularly on guard against exposure to the things that you know trigger your allergies. Also, during this period, consider using immune system enhancers sold in most health food stores.

ALZHEIMER'S DISEASE

(Channeled by Ignatious)

Alzheimer's disease is a disease that attacks people in their middle and later years. It is a form of senility, and not much progress has yet been made in its understanding or treatment. What we do know is that it is a degenerative disease destroying its victims' mental and physical capabilities.

Also, as this disease is caused by an unknown source, possibly an organism, it is wise to work with the Deva in charge of the organism involved with Alzheimer's disease (see Chapter VI on the Devic Kingdom). After a contact is made, ask the Deva to remove the organism which may be causing the disease, out of the Physical Body and the Etheric Body as well.

Then ask the Etheric Body to work with the brain to repair and restore memory connections using the Ketheric Template (7th layer of the Aura) as a blueprint for what the proper memory connections and a healthy brain should be.

Ask the Etheric Body to have the brain make new connections as needed. Repeat this procedure often.

Then ask the Etheric Body to remove the Miasm for Alzheimer's disease from the Base Chakra (#1). Repeat this request until the Miasm has been removed.

Regularly ask the Etheric Body to clear the Mental Body several times a week until progress is noted. Then do this less often.

Ask the Etheric Body on a regular basis to keep the Third Eye Chakra (#6) and the Base Chakra (#1) unblocked, clear, and balanced.

This is an illness where Bio-Etheric Healing has a chance of working better when it is caught very early.

ANEMIA

This is a condition where the quality or quantity of the blood supply is deficient. There are many factors which are involved in causing this condition, including the proper functioning of the body to produce new blood cells, as well as dietary factors which provide the body's nutritional needs. Anemia is characterized by an excessive tiredness, debilitation, and complete lack of energy.

Anemia most directly involves the Throat Chakra (#5) and the Spleen Chakra and their vortices which may be malfunctioning.

First, ask the Etheric Body for each of these two chakras to find out if each or both are involved. Then for the chakra(s) or their vortices which are involved, ask the Etheric Body if the problem is one of needed repair, blockage, cloudiness, or an imbalance. After that, ask the Etheric Body to repair, break up blocked energy, clear up or balance the implicated chakra(s) and their vortices, as needed.

ANGINA PECTORIS

Broadly speaking, this condition in nearly all cases involves an imbalance of the blood circulation between the extremities of the body and the blood circulation going to the central parts and internal organs. This lack of proper balance creates many often severe problems in the functioning of the various body organs and the brain due to under-supply or over-supply of blood.

Ask the Etheric Body to determine where there is an imbalance to the flow of blood in the body by referring to the 7th layer of the Aura, the Ketheric Template, to determine what the proper flow of blood should be like. Then ask it to correct the imbalance as soon as possible.

Angina pectoris may involve an underactive Heart Chakra (#4). First, ask the Etheric Body to see if that is the case. If so, ask the Etheric Body to balance the Heart Chakra and its vortices. Repeat as necessary.

It is also necessary to ask the Etheric Body if this condition is caused by the Anxiety/Fear Syndrome. If that is so, follow directions for Anxiety/Fear, as well.

ANXIETY/FEAR

Anxiety is a mental state of painful uneasiness over an impending or anticipated event, real or imagined. Sometimes it is a result of nonspecific, generalized fear. Anxiety can trigger reactions in the body such as unusual chemical activity, and also interfere with the body's normal and necessary activities. It can result in problems such as ulcers, migraines, rheumatoid arthritis, colitis, asthma, and other physical ailments. It is wise to consult a medical professional, especially one with psychological training for treatment of anxiety.

At the same time, regardless of its cause or physical result, anxiety always causes blockage of the Heart Chakra (#4), thus lending itself readily to the possibility of Bio-Etheric Healing. Therefore, in addition to professional psychological attention, it can be very helpful to ask the Etheric Body to clear the blockage of the Heart Chakra and its vortices.

Sometimes the anxiety may be caused by Karma or Traumas of past lives or present lives. Check with the Etheric Body if this is the case. Clearing these from the Aura may be helpful in resolving the situation. (See sections on Karma and Traumas.) It is also suggested that you ask the Etheric Body to clear the Emotional Body of anxieties that arise in the present. This precaution is especially useful when a person has been conditioned to respond to particular situations with anxiety.

ARTHRITIS
(See Osteoarthritis and Rheumatoid Arthritis)

ASTHMA
Asthma is a debilitating disease because it affects the lungs and one's ability to breathe. Therefore, life is dependent upon being able to deal with this disease effectively.

Anxiety and fear are often overlooked causes of this disease. (See separate listing, Anxiety/Fear, for further information and help.)

Allergies are also the culprit in some asthma cases, especially allergies due to toxins in the air. (See separate listing, Allergies.)

Asthmatic attacks may also involve the Throat Chakra (#5). Chakra damage or damage to its vortices may be due to sudden emotional shock which can initiate asthmatic attacks causing injury to the vortices or the chakra. Ask the Etheric Body to repair this chakra and its vortices, to break up any blocked energy, and/or to clear and balance the chakra and vortices as needed.

AUTO-IMMUNE SYSTEM PROBLEMS

Auto-immune system problems may be triggered by anxiety and fear from one's current or past life Traumas. This can lead to a blockage of the Heart Chakra (#4) and/or its vortices. Also, an imbalance or cloudiness of the Heart Chakra and vortices may be involved. Karma may also be implicated.

Ask the Etheric Body to ascertain which of these problems with the Heart Chakra or vortices is involved. Then ask the Etheric Body to break up any blocked energy, or to clear or balance the chakra and vortices as needed. Repeat as necessary.

Ask the Etheric Body whether Karma or Traumas are involved. If so, see separate listings on each and treat accordingly.

BLOOD DISORDERS

Hemophilia
(Channeled by Kwan Yin)

Ask the Etheric Body to repair or create anew the cells involved with the clotting of blood using the Ketheric Template (7th layer of the Aura), as a guide. Ask the Etheric Body to create and multiply cells in the amount needed for the whole body. Sitting in an upright position so that you do not fall asleep, you can repeat the procedure each night or every other night until there is improvement. It will probably take between one and one-and-a-half years to notice improvement.

Hypertension — High Blood Pressure

Difficulties with blood pressure may involve the Crown Chakra (#7), the Third Eye Chakra (#6), the Throat Chakra (#5), the Heart Chakra (#4), and the Alta Major Chakra. Using Communication Skills, ask the Etheric Body to identify the problem and which chakra or combination of chakras is involved. Then ask the Etheric Body to repair the chakra(s) and vortices, to break up any blocked energy, and to clear and balance the chakra(s) and vortices as needed.

You can also ask your Etheric Body to normalize the blood pressure. When the Emotional Body is involved due to anxiety of having your blood pressure measured, ask the Etheric Body to clear the Emotional Body first and to provide you with a normal reading. You may have to repeat this procedure often.

It is possible that Trauma and Karma may be involved in hypertension. (See separate listings on each.)

Idiopathic Thrombocyte Penia — ITP
(Channeled by Kwan Yin)

A low blood platelet count in the Physical Body with a cause of unknown origin is called idiopathic thrombocyte penia— ITP. It may involve a blocked or damaged Spleen Chakra. Use Communication Skills to test the Etheric Body for confirmation. If the test is positive, then ask the Etheric Body to break up the blocked energy or repair the Spleen Chakra, whichever is necessary.

It is also possible that there is some defect in the cell structure of the platelet. Ask the Etheric Body if that may be a factor in this problem. If the answer is "yes," ask the Etheric Body to compare the cellular structure of the platelet with what the proper cellular structure should be, using the 7th layer of the Aura, the Ketheric Template layer, as a guide. Then tell the Etheric Body to make the necessary changes to correct the cellular structure.

White Cell Deficiency

The spleen manufactures white cells and stores iron. White blood cells combat infection. During infections, the spleen manufactures more white blood cells for this important purpose, and so its proper functioning is critical. The Spleen Chakra is directly involved in the health of the spleen and is also related to the platelet count in the blood.

In the case of white cell deficiency, the problem may be related to a blocked, cloudy, unbalanced, or damaged Spleen Chakra or its vortices. Ask the Etheric Body for each of these four potential factors, individually, if they are part of the problem with the chakra or its vortices. Then for each of the factors which are implicated, ask the Etheric Body to unblock, clear, balance, or repair the chakra and its vortices accordingly.

BONE-RELATED PROBLEMS
(See also Osteoarthritis and Rheumatoid Arthritis)

Poor calcium metabolism is a factor in many bone-related health problems. These include arthritis (both rheumatoid and osteo), osteoporosis, bone loss in the teeth, and fragility of the body's bones.

Maintaining the strength and health of our bone structure at all stages of life requires two things:

1. The proper amount of calcium/magnesium taken in by the body
2. The proper metabolism of the calcium/magnesium to insure the utilization of these elements by the body.

Poor calcium/magnesium metabolism is very often due to an imbalance of the alkaline/acid ratio in the body. Adding more acidity to our body can help fight degenerative bone diseases and increase the absorption of calcium/magnesium. However, intake of sugars and white flour products inhibit the absorption of calcium/magnesium by the body, and thus encourages degenerative bone diseases.

Calcium metabolism often involves the Throat Chakra (#5) which must be balanced for normal calcium metabolism. If you have problems metabolizing calcium, check the Etheric Body to see if the problem is due to an imbalance in this chakra. If so, ask the Etheric Body to create the proper balance. Also, check to see if the chakra is cloudy, blocked, or damaged, and ask the Etheric Body to make the appropriate repair.

Also, if you have a specific problem which has been diagnosed by your health professional as rheumatoid or osteoarthritis, osteoporosis, or bone loss in teeth, refer to the section on each of these individual problems for further information.

BRAIN-INVOLVED PROBLEMS
(Channeled by Kwan Yin)

There are many specific health complaints related to the brain. Several are covered here. Generally, the Crown Chakra (#7) and the Third Eye Chakra (#6) are involved. The pineal gland may also be involved. The Crown Chakra usually is related to functions covered by the upper part of the brain and the right eye. The Third Eye Chakra may relate mostly to issues of the lower brain and left eye. In working with the chakras in brain-related issues, be very careful not to overstimulate the chakras, as this may induce mental problems.

Dyslexia

Ask the Etheric Body to work with the brain to correct the imbalance of the brain cells in the area involved in dyslexia (which can differ from person to person). Ask the Etheric Body to correct any malfunction of the circuits of the brain, using the Ketheric Template (7th layer of the Aura) as a blueprint for the proper circuitry.

Repeat this procedure often, especially at the beginning, about every day for one or more months. Then cut this back to four times a week for three or four months, and once a week after that until the dyslexia is corrected. After that, it may be necessary to do the procedure once a month for a year or so to prevent any regression.

In the case of learning disabilities, this problem is handled the same way as dyslexia, but you must substitute the words "learning disabilities" for the word "dyslexia" in your request of the Etheric Body. Follow the same instructions.

Epilepsy

Epilepsy involves a malfunction of the brain cells. Ask the Etheric Body to work closely with the Ketheric Template of the Aura (7th layer) to heal the cells of the brain that are malfunctioning and causing the epilepsy. If it cannot heal the cells because they are too badly damaged, ask the Etheric Body to replace those cells with normal cells. Repeat this procedure every night to start, or as close to that as possible. New cells may take one and one-half to two years to be regenerated, while repairing cells takes less time.

Memory Loss

Memory loss often occurs with the deterioration or loss of function of certain brain cells and/or connections of the neurons specializing in the process of memory. This may occur as a natural result of aging or sometimes as a result of disease.

It may be possible to offset or limit the memory loss by asking the Etheric Body to rebuild the connections and to create new cells where necessary. Ask the Etheric Body to do so by using the Ketheric Template (7th layer of the Aura) as a blueprint indicating what a healthy brain with proper memory connections and cells originally possessed, and to try to recreate that. This request needs to be repeated on a regular basis and any improvement will take time.

CANCER
(Channeled by Kwan Yin)

Cancer is one of the most complex and difficult illnesses to work with. Although there is knowledge about the process of cancerous cell growth, there is not yet enough knowledge about "how" the process starts or, more importantly, "why." Aside from external environmental and chemical causes, one of the contributing factors may be of a psychological nature which triggers or impedes certain chemical or physical activities of the body. Regardless, all of the external factors, as well as any psychological ones, may have affected the health of the Aura and the Chakra System.

Bio-Etheric Healing deals specifically with the health of the Aura and the Chakra System to affect the health of the Physical Body and help it to get well. Thus, it can be used as a support system for a person undergoing surgery, chemotherapy, and radiation for cancer. Bio-Etheric Healing has a greater chance for helping when the disease is caught in its early stages. Although the cancerous cells, themselves, may be in a different part of the body, the disease most often makes itself evident first at the solar plexus level of the Aura. Unresolved psychological problems often cause blockage of the energy in the Base Chakra (#1), and an imbalance as well. This is true of the Solar Plexus Chakra (#3) also.

However, psychological problems may be a result of Traumas of past or present lives, and these, too, may be related to the cancer, and causing malfunctioning of the Chakra System. It is also possible that Karma can induce problems resulting in cancer. As both Traumas and Karma related to the particular cancer may be implicated and causing malfunction of the Chakra System, these possibilities need to be explored, and if confirmed, dealt with in Bio-Etheric Healing.

This involved situation, then, calls for a series of steps, as follows:

- First, it is wise to get the Miasm of cancer out of the Base Chakra. (See section on Miasms.) Using your Communication Skills, ask your Etheric Body to remove the Miasm of cancer from the Base Chakra.
- Next, ask the Etheric Body if the Base Chakra or its vortices is blocked, out of balance, cloudy or damaged. If any of these conditions exist, ask the Etheric Body to carry out the needed

treatment; that is, to unblock, balance, clear, or repair the chakra and/or its vortices.

- After that, the Solar Plexus Chakra and its vortices, which are of great importance to work with cancer, must be explored in the same way. Follow the exact same procedure for this chakra as described in the preceding paragraph to restore its health.

- Beside the two previously mentioned chakras critical to work with cancer, this disease can be affected by and, in turn, affect the other chakras because of the cancer's physical location in the body. Therefore, it is advisable to check the other five main chakras and their vortices, individually, to see if any of them need attention. If so, follow the exact same procedures, asking the Etheric Body if there is blockage, imbalance, cloudiness, or damage, and asking it to do the appropriate repair work.

- Now it is important to ask the Etheric Body if any Traumas related to the specific cancer are involved. Do so separately for Traumas of present as well as past lives. If any Trauma(s) are implicated in the illness, ask the Etheric Body for each one separately, to remove them from the Mental Body. However, before doing so, you must first ask permission of the Soul for removal of any such Trauma(s) related to the cancer. (See section on Traumas.)

- As there are multiple past lives, the possibility exists for more than one such Trauma to be involved. Therefore, it is wise to ask the Etheric Body again about the existence of any other such Trauma.

- To determine if Karma is involved with the cancer, ask the Etheric Body directly. If there is an affirmative answer, ask the Etheric Body to remove the Karma involved in the illness out of the outer layers of the Aura.

- Then ask the Etheric Body to use the 5th layer of the Aura (which consists of negative space) to make room in this 5th layer for the removal of the cancer. Ask the Etheric Body to use the Ketheric Template (the 7th layer of the Aura) to serve as a blueprint of what a healthy body with no cancer looks like, and thus, to dissolve the cancer accordingly from the Aura. The Physical Body's cancer may then dissolve because its roots in the Aura are gone.

- As a preventative against future cancer cell growth, ask the Etheric Body on a periodic basis to kill any new cancer cells that appear at the Etheric Level, thus preventing them from reaching the Physical Body.
- Chemotherapy and radiation can damage or destroy the fragile Aura and its outside web. Ask the Etheric Body to strengthen the outside web of the Aura and repair the damaged areas.
- The Spleen Chakra, although not one of the seven main chakras, is important in working with cancer, particular during chemotherapy treatments. The Spleen Chakra is involved in the production of white blood cells which are damaged and destroyed in chemotherapy. It must be kept unblocked. Ask the Etheric Body if the Spleen Chakra is blocked. If so, ask the Etheric Body to unblock it. Do so periodically after each chemotherapy treatment to keep it open and working properly providing the proper flow and level of critical white blood cells. Should the white blood cell count fall below the normal level, ask the Etheric Body to increase their production to achieve normalcy.

Cautionary Note: At all times, be aware not to ask the Etheric Body to work on more than one procedure at a time, so as not to deplete the body's energy level too seriously. Also, be aware that it may be necessary to repeat some of these procedures as necessary to accomplish their individual goals. You can ask the Etheric Body whether a goal has been accomplished or if repetition is required.

All the above suggestions are as support procedures to be used as an adjunct to a medical program or alternative medical program for the treatment of cancer. At the same time, it may be possible that these same procedures can help reduce or remove some types of very slow-growing cancers. In this process, there is a possibility that some minor bleeding may occur as a medium for eliminating these cancer cells.

CHILDHOOD DISEASES

From early infancy, children can respond very readily to Bio-Etheric Healing work. The child's Etheric Body is spirit that has lived many lifetimes and is able to communicate with you even when the Physical Body is very new to this world. Therefore, one may be able to relieve a small child's discomfort via the use of Bio-Etheric Healing techniques.

Please be sure not to ask for more than one request for healing at a time. You don't want to incur any problems for a child by asking his Etheric Body for more than it, or the child's Physical Body can handle at one time.

Chickenpox

Ask the Etheric Body to destroy the virus and to dry up the pustules and make sure no more appear. If there is pain, ask the Etheric Body to dissolve the blocked energy affecting the area. Repeat if necessary.

Childhood Infections: Colds, Earaches, Sore Throat

At the first sign of any infection coming on, or as a preventative measure if you feel that the child has been exposed to someone else's infection, it is wise to ask the child's Etheric Body to kill any bacteria or virus at the Etheric Level before they reach the Physical Body.

If the infection has already caught hold, ask the Etheric Body to kill the bacteria or virus that is causing the infection. Name the site of the infection. If there is pain associated with this, ask the Etheric Body for the blocked energy to be released and be specific regarding the location of the pain.

Colic

Colic is sometimes related to damage of the Chakra System due to the birth process. It can also be due to blocked energy. It may require clearing of the Solar Plexus Chakra (#3) and/or the Sacral Chakra (#2) or their vortices. Ask the Etheric Body to heal any damage to the Chakra System and to clear and break up any blocked energy involved in the pain.

Colic may also be related to slow development of the digestive system. Therefore, you can ask the Etheric Body to speed up this development to reach its proper stage of maturity.

Irritability
(Channeled by Ignatious)

Children under three years old sometimes get fragments of their mother's Astral Body into their own Astral Body during the birth process. This can cause crying and irritability. You can ask the baby's Etheric Body individually to clear the Astral Body, Mental Body, and the Emotional Body.

Gas Pain

If the child's pain seems to be gas related, check this by asking its Etheric Body if it is gas causing the pain. If so, then ask its Etheric Body to break up the blocked energy causing the gas pain.

Teething Pain

Ask the Etheric Body of the child to knock out blocked energy causing teething pain. This may help to diminish or take away the pain of teething. Repeat as necessary. Also, ask the Etheric Body to have the Physical Body create the necessary endorphins to provide a natural anesthetic for the child.

Sometimes, during the teething process, a child's Throat Chakra (#5) gets cloudy, causing discomfort for the child. Ask the Etheric Body of the child to remove the cloudiness of the Throat Chakra and to continue doing so as necessary. It will make the child more comfortable.

Thrush

Thrush is a fungus, and as a lower life form, it is governed by the Devic Kingdom. (See Chapter VI, "The Devic Kingdom and its Role in Bio-Etheric Healing.")

The mother needs to ask the Deva of the Candida fungus to get the fungus out of the affected child's body. If an infant's fungus has been contracted from the mother during breast feeding, the Deva of the Candida fungus should be asked to remove this fungus from the mother's body as well. Repeat once a week until clear.

CHOLESTEROL PROBLEMS

Ask the Etheric Body to lower the cholesterol level. You will need to tell the Etheric Body what you would like the cholesterol level to be. Be realistic.

CHRONIC FATIGUE SYNDROME

Treat the same as for Epstein-Barr Syndrome.

CIRCULATORY SYSTEM PROBLEMS

Problems of the circulatory system may be due to an unbalanced Heart Chakra (#4) and/or vortices. Check the Etheric Body to verify. Ask the Etheric Body to balance or repair this chakra and its vortices, to break up any blocked energy and to clear the chakra and vortices as needed. Repeat as necessary.

CLAUSTROPHOBIA
(Channeled by Kwan Yin)

This is a morbid dread of being in closed rooms or narrow spaces. The origin of this fear is usually unknown. Traumas of past lives or one's present life, as well as Karma, may be implicated. Bio-Etheric Healing may be very effective in dealing with this problem.

To work with claustrophobia, check the Etheric Body to see if Traumas or Karma is involved. If either is implicated, please refer to listings under Anxiety/Fear or under Traumas, or under Karma, as appropriate, before proceeding.

COLDS — BACTERIAL OR VIRAL

At the very first sign of a cold, check the Etheric Body to see if it is being caused by detoxification for a previous problem, or a real cold.

If it is a real cold, ask the Etheric Body to remove it from the body, whether it is bacterial or viral. Tell the Etheric Body where the infection seems to be. Repeat again, and again, if necessary.

If the cold is not caught at its first signs, you may have cold symptoms, but they will most likely be much less severe than usual. However, if you have a stuffed nose, you can ask the Etheric Body to break up the blocked energy of the Third Eye Chakra (#6), to clear the nose. If you have a sore throat, or a cough, you can ask the Etheric Body to break up the blocked energy and clear the Throat Chakra (#5) for some relief. If you have phlegm, ask your Etheric Body to dissolve it. You can repeat these requests as often as you feel you need to.

For additional help, you may provide your body with nutritional support. Take one-half or a full gram of vitamin C and 500 milligrams of chelated zinc once or twice a day, as needed.

COLITIS

(Channeled by Kwan Yin)

Colitis results from two basic causes; namely, a dysfunction of the immune system and by fear, which in turn, causes blockage of the Heart Chakra (#4) and its vortices. A blocked Heart Chakra is involved with the bleeding in colitis.

In addition to these two factors, Karma may sometimes be involved. If Karma is involved, it works as an overriding factor and must first be removed from the two outer layers of the Aura before any other treatment is applied. (See specific listing for Karma Related to Illness.)

In working with the immune system, ask the Etheric Body to correct any malfunctioning in the place where it is occurring. Then ask the Etheric Body to break up any blocked energy in the Heart Chakra and its vortices and clear them. Ask the Etheric Body to remove the Miasm of colitis out of the body in order to lessen the chance of colitis recurring.

In dealing with the fear aspect of colitis, one should first explore the basic cause of the fear with a medical professional. While this exploration is taking place, you can control the bleeding in colitis by using cayenne pepper capsules, about eight or nine a day at 40,000 HU strength each. Take less after the bleeding stops, but reduce the dosage slowly. Use Communication Skills to check how much cayenne you need to take regularly. If bleeding starts again, resume use of cayenne pepper.

To help heal internal scar tissue, start with 400 IU's of vitamin E and build up slowly to 800 IU's over a several-week period. Use your Communication Skills to determine the amount your body can tolerate safely.

To treat colitis caused by fear, you must remove Trauma of fear from the Aura if it is allowed by the Soul. Ask the Soul for permission. The Soul may not allow removal of the Trauma in cases where the Trauma acts as a safety net to prevent a person from having a life-threatening experience.

If you are told that you can go ahead to remove the Trauma, first find out if it is from the current life and/or from past life(s). Then ask your Etheric Body to remove the Trauma(s) from the Aura. You may need to get the Traumas of past lives out of the Aura before clearing the Traumas of the current life out of the Aura. Clear the Emotional Body as well to complete the therapy. Clearing the Emotional Body may need to be done as often as needed after bouts of anxiety. (See listings for Anxiety/Fear and also Traumas.)

Note: Keep in mind not to overload the Etheric Body with more than two requests simultaneously, because this may seriously deplete the energy level of the Physical Body. Also, be aware that detoxification symptoms, such as colds, rash, et cetera, will probably result from this work.

EARACHE

An earache caused by infection involves the Third Eye Chakra (#6). Ask the Etheric Body to clear the blocked energy in the chakra and vortices causing the pain. Ask the Etheric Body to knock out any infection whether it is viral or bacterial. Repeat if necessary.

EPSTEIN-BARR SYNDROME

(Channeled by Kwan Yin)

Epstein-Barr Syndrome is a disease caused by a virus of the herpes family. It affects the body's immune system and can cause other serious infections and complications. This disease also causes a major loss of the body's energy. As the Chakra System is the means for distributing energy throughout the body, all chakras are affected. However, the Base Chakra (#1), the Solar Plexus Chakra (#3), the Throat Chakra (#5), and the Crown Chakra (#7) seem to be of primary importance in this disorder.

Karma may also be involved in this ailment. If so, as the influence of Karma is primary, it may limit the progress of any healing and must first be removed from the two outer layers of the Aura. Therefore, you must use your Communication Skills to determine if Karma is involved in this situation. If it is playing a role, ask the Etheric Body to remove the Karma involved from the outer two layers of the Aura. This action can take two weeks or so, and you can check the Etheric Body to see if it has been accomplished.

Then ask the Etheric Body which of the chakras are involved in your particular situation. After determining which chakras are involved from those itemized above, proceed to make the appropriate request(s) of your Etheric Body in terms of remedial action.

For each chakra involved, ask if the chakra and its vortices are unbalanced, blocked or cloudy. For those chakras or their vortices that need treatment, ask the Etheric Body to provide the appropriate work of either balancing, unblocking or clearing them. As work with Epstein-Barr Syndrome is more complex, it requires these additional remedial procedures:

- To limit and reduce the possible harm to the body's immune system, it is wise to remove the virus from the body as soon as possible. To accomplish this most efficiently, work directly with the Deva of the Epstein-Barr Syndrome organism. Call for the Deva and ask it to get this organism out of the Physical and Etheric Body. (See Chapter VI on the Devic Kingdom.)
- The immune system will need strengthening. Ask the Etheric Body to heal and strengthen it.
- It may be particularly useful to call upon the spirit source of The White Healing Light to help heal the immune system and hasten the rate of recovery. (See Chapter V under Other Energy Sources.)
- Ask the Etheric Body to remove the Miasm for Epstein-Barr Syndrome from the Base Chakra (#1).
- Ask the Etheric Body to strengthen and normalize the adrenal gland to restore the energy level to the Physical Body.
- Ask the Etheric Body to get the digestive system functioning properly to convert food into energy.
- Ask the Etheric Body to increase the vibrational rate of the Physical Body for it to function at an optimal level.

Additionally, the following suggestions may be helpful in these specific cases:

- If pain is involved, ask the Etheric Body to break up the blocked energy causing the pain, specifying the exact location of the pain. Repeat as often as necessary.
- Ask your Etheric Body if Traumas of past or present lives are involved. If the answer is "yes," refer to the listing on Traumas for specific instructions.
- It is possible that parasites in the intestine or elsewhere in the body are present with this disease. Check with the Etheric Body to see if this is so. If yes, then see the separate listing in this chapter on Intestinal Parasites.

It may be necessary, especially in remedial work with the chakras, to repeat the requests to the Etheric Body at intervals. You may consult the Etheric Body on the need for repetition.

Finally, it is important not to overload the Etheric Body with more than two requests simultaneously because of the danger of depleting the Physical Body's energy level.

For nutritional support, eat high protein foods. Do not eat sugar or white flour products. Take strong multivitamins, including B complex, C, D, E, A, and calcium/magnesium in the amounts the body needs. Inquire as to what the Physical Body needs using Communication Skills. Monitor the progress at intervals. Maximal adrenal gland drops may help, or use any other type of adrenal gland supplement. You may also use immune system enhancers sold at most health food stores.

EYE-RELATED PROBLEMS

The right eye is governed by the Crown Chakra (#7) and the left eye is governed by the Third Eye Chakra (#6). In problems with either eye, you must address the corresponding chakra involved. Ask the Etheric Body to clear the chakras and vortices. Also ask the Etheric Body to unblock the chakras and their vortices and to repair any damage as needed.

Color Blindness

It may be possible to help color blindness. However, this could take one and one-half to two years before improvement is noticed when the brain cells related to it are damaged. Replacing missing cells may be possible, but that will take longer or may be difficult to achieve at best, without constant repetition of the suggestions provided here.

Ask the Etheric Body to repair any damaged cells that may be causing the problem or to create missing cells, if that is necessary. Ask the person's brain to help in the process. Ask the Etheric Body to work with the Ketheric Template (7th layer of the Aura) as a blueprint of what healthy brain cells should look like in order to do this repair or to create new cells. It is important to repeat these procedures at intervals.

Vision Problems

It may be possible to help vision problems such as near or far-sightedness and astigmatism. Ask the Etheric Body to correct the particular condition using the Ketheric Template (7th layer of the Aura) as a blueprint of the eye in normal vision. This process works very slowly and it is advisable to repeat this procedure at regular intervals.

Dry Eye Syndrome

Ask the Etheric Body to lubricate the eyes and it will do so.

FATIGUE

Fatigue may be an indicator of illness, nervous exhaustion, or emotional stress. It may also relate to the state of the chakras or the function of the adrenal gland. The chakras involved are the Throat Chakra (#5) and the Base Chakra (#1).

Ask the Etheric Body if either of these two chakras are involved. For the chakra(s) that is involved, ask the Etheric Body to break up any blocked energy in that chakra and its vortices, and if it is cloudy, to clear up that cloudiness, also. Then, ask the Etheric Body individually, for each chakra that is involved, to balance it and its vortices.

For the adrenal gland, ask the Etheric Body to normalize its activity and to repair any malfunction, as required.

For fatigue due to stress, see separate listing under Stress.

FEET PROBLEMS

The main chakra related to the feet is the Base Chakra (#1). For weak arches, ask the Etheric Body to strengthen the arches. For Achilles tendon pain, ask the Etheric Body to break up blocked energy affecting the tendon. For pain anywhere on the foot, ask the Etheric Body to break up blocked energy affecting that area. For infection, ask the Etheric Body to remove the infection. For athlete's foot, see listing for Fungus. For neuromas, see listing for Neuromas.

FLU

Ask the Etheric Body to remove the flu virus out of your body. Do this at the first sign of infection for best results. If the flu is in the body for several days, you need to repeat this procedure often.

For additional help, you may provide your body with nutritional support. Take one-half or a full gram of vitamin C and 500 milligrams of chelated zinc once or twice a day, as needed.

FREE RADICAL — OXIDANTS

(Problems Related to Presence of)

In the normal functioning of the body, the process of converting the oxygen, liquids, and food we consume into the energy we need to function, sometimes produces stray chemicals called "free radicals" or "oxidants."

These free radical/oxidants are a destructive force in the body attacking other important and necessary healthy cells. Free radicals play a significant role in the deterioration of the cardiovascular system and the central nervous system, and may be significantly involved in the formation of neuritic plaques associated with senile dementia of the Alzheimer type. They also destroy norepinephrine in the body, the reduction of which is associated with aging, formation of wrinkles, and depression. Arthritis, formation of tumors, and cell loss in the body also are problems in which free radicals are suspect.

Products called "anti-oxidants" which come in several forms, including tablets, are usually employed by medical practitioners to rid the body of free radicals. Bio-Etheric Healing suggests that it may be possible to remove these free radicals by asking the Etheric Body to rid the Physical Body of these rogue oxidants. You can ask the Etheric Body to remove these free radical oxidants out of the body. It is wise to make this request on a periodic basis.

FUNGUS — ATHLETE'S FOOT

As a lower life form, the fungus of athlete's foot is governed by the Devic Kingdom. (See Chapter VI, "The Devic Kingdom and its Role in Bio-Etheric Healing.") Therefore, it is necessary to call forth the Deva of the athlete's foot fungus, using your Communication Skills. Talk to the Deva. Be friendly but polite. Ask her to take the fungus out of your body. It will take time. Talk to the

Deva at intervals to keep her working for you in getting rid of the fungus. Ask the Etheric Body to calm the feet at night.

GROWTHS — (NON-CANCEROUS)

All growths begin in the Aura at the Etheric Body level before they materialize in the Physical Body. They must be removed there first before they can disappear from the Physical Body. You can ask your Etheric Body to get the growth out of the Aura. To accomplish this, you must also ask your Etheric Body to work with the Etheric Template (5th layer of the Aura) which is in negative space to make room for the growth to be removed. (See section on the layers of the Aura in Chapter II for further explanation.)

After this is done, ask your Etheric Body to work with the Ketheric Template (7th layer of the Aura) which is a blueprint of the body and to use it as a guide to locate the growth (which will be revealed by the template to be extraneous) and to remove it.

Finally, as the Solar Plexus Chakra (#3) and its vortices are involved in growths in the body, it is necessary to ask the Etheric Body to balance this chakra and its vortices.

Once the root of the growth is removed from the Aura, the physical counterpart takes a long time to be reabsorbed by the Physical Body and disappear. At this point, if you choose to have physical surgery, you will know that the Auric root of the growth is gone. If you do have physical surgery first, the Aura will still have the growth in it. Recovery will be faster and better if you remove the growth from the Aura as well.

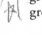

HAIR LOSS

It may be possible to stimulate new hair growth. Ask the Etheric Body to make your hair grow back (specify where). This may take two or three years before you notice anything. It does not hurt to repeat the request every once in a while. If the hair is now naturally gray, you can specify that the color of the new growth come in with its original color.

HAY FEVER

Hay fever is related to the Third Eye Chakra (#6). Ask the Etheric Body to balance the 6th Chakra and vortices and to clear the blocked energy. Repeat as necessary. (Also see listing on Allergies.)

HEARING LOSS
(Channeled by Kwan Yin)

Hearing loss may sometimes involve blocked energy in the Chakra System. The Alta Major Chakra, or the Third Eye Chakra (#6) may be involved. Ask the Etheric Body to confirm if either of these chakras or their vortices are blocked. If confirmed, ask the Etheric Body to break up the blockage involved in the hearing loss.

Hearing loss can also involve nerve damage. As channeled by Kwan Yin, it may be possible to repair the damaged nerve that relates to hearing loss. Ask the Etheric Body to repair the nerve damage related to hearing loss by using the Ketheric Template (7th Layer of the Aura) as a blueprint of what a healthy nerve should be. Do this every night or every morning and continue this until you can notice improvement. You can then do this less often as the improvement continues.

HEART DISEASE/PROBLEMS
Coronary Heart Disease
(Channeled by Kwan Yin)

Coronary heart disease may be due to an underactive Heart Chakra (#4) which causes it to be out of balance. Ask the Etheric Body to balance this chakra and its vortices. Repeat as necessary.

Hardening of the Arteries
(Channeled by Kwan Yin)

For hardening of the arteries, or blocked arteries, work with the Etheric Body. Ask the Etheric Body to clear the arteries of all plaque and any other substances that would interfere with the free flow of blood to and from the heart and to dispose of that matter in the normal way. Do this every night before falling asleep as prevention. It may be very effective to prevent a heart attack due to blockage of the normal flow of blood. If you miss a day here and there, it is no problem, but continue this program to maintain healthy blood flow.

Missing Heartbeats (A Type of Arrhythmia)

There is a general classification of heartbeat irregularities that are known as arrhythmia. These include missing heartbeats, rapid heartbeats, etc. Bio-Etheric healing may be of value with the problem of missing heartbeats.

Missing heartbeats can be the result of a blocked Heart Chakra (#4) or the result of a damaged Heart Chakra. In either case, there is major interference with the normal flow of energy through this important junction of the Etheric Body. Both of these types of problems should be investigated by questions posed to the Etheric Body.

For a damaged chakra, please ask the Etheric Body to heal the damaged chakra.

For a blocked Heart Chakra, ask the Etheric Body to break up the blocked energy of the Heart Chakra and its vortices. You may need to repeat this as often as necessary.

To the person experiencing missing heartbeats, the awareness of this interruption in such an important muscle function can cause understandable anxiety and fear. As anxiety and fear by themselves can also cause blockage of the Heart Chakra, one thing can lead to the other. Therefore, it is critical to investigate whether anxiety and fear are involved in the blockage of the Heart Chakra, and to address those situations as well. (See listing under Anxiety/Fear and follow those directions also.)

HEPATITIS

(See Infectious Hepatitis)

HIATAL HERNIA

Hiatal Hernia is sometimes related to a damaged Throat Chakra (#5). Use your Communication Skills to ask the Etheric Body if the chakra is damaged. If so, ask the Etheric Body to repair the 5th Chakra and any of its vortices that are involved using the Ketheric Template (7th Layer of the Aura) as a guide for this repair. Repeat as necessary.

HIV VIRUS (POSITIVE)

(Channeled by Ignatious)

This disease is extremely complex and continues to confound medical science. Progress in healing, if at all possible, is difficult and extremely slow. Even if one succeeds to get the virus out of the body, it would only represent the beginning, because this disease causes so much damage that much more healing work still needs to be accomplished. Also, one must be in constant contact with his or her healing professional to face and deal with any new problems that are likely to arise because of the damage to the body, particularly to the immune system. Remember, that the earlier the treatment is started, the better.

Bio-Etheric Healing work with the HIV virus requires communication with the Devic Kingdom. Please refer to Chapter VI on the Devic Kingdom before proceeding to work on this disease.

There are two phases to this healing work. First, is the work with the Deva of the HIV virus. Second, is working with the Etheric Body of the individual involved.

To start, use your Communication Skills (Inner Speaking/ Inner Listening) to ask for the Deva of the HIV virus. If you are not able to receive a thought response, you can still contact the Deva, using Inner Speaking, but use Kinesiology, Head Motions or Radiesthesia to get a response. Ask the Deva to remove the virus out of the body (provide name and address of the person to be healed). If the Deva agrees to do so, then ask her to kill the virus. This part may take two days, or weeks, or months, or years, depending on a variety of factors involving the patient and his health condition. It may be necessary to repeat this entire procedure on a monthly basis, as needed. [Subsequent to this message from Ignatious, Kwan Yin has channeled that it is wise to check the Etheric Body of the person involved once a month to see if the virus was still in the body. She also felt that contacting the Deva of the HIV Virus about once a month to ask about the progress in eliminating the virus was appropriate.]

After working with the Deva, ask the Etheric Body of the person involved to clear the Base Chakra (#1) and the Sacral Chakra (#2) and their vortices. Also ask the Etheric Body to break up any blocked energy in these chakras and their vortices and to balance them. Sometimes other chakras are involved and so you must ask the Etheric Body if this is so, and ask for these chakras to be treated also. Be sure not to omit the Spleen Chakra and the Alta Major Chakra in this inquiry.

It is important also to ask the Etheric Body to strengthen the immune system and ask it to heal the problems caused by the HIV virus. One such problem is a serious reduction of the "T cells" in the body. Therefore, it is wise to ask the Etheric Body daily to restore the "T cell" level to that of a healthy person.

Another problem is the danger from CMV (cytomegalovirus), a virus in the herpes family which exists in a major portion of the population, but is held in check by a healthy immune system. With an immune system weakened by the HIV virus, the CMV herpes virus can flourish and attack various organs of the body and reach the retina of the eye causing serious damage and even blindness. Ask the Etheric Body to destroy the CMV herpes virus wherever it may be in the body. Then, be sure to ask the Etheric Body to get the Miasm of the CMV herpes virus out of the Base Chakra (#1).

Remember to make requests of the Etheric Body for healing help with these problems, individually, being careful not to overload the Etheric Body with too many requests at the same time. Space this work so as not to deplete the Physical Body of energy, but repeat the requests at regular intervals.

It is important to remember here, as in all healing work, that a process of detoxification will probably occur, which may manifest itself in a variety of ways, including extreme tiredness, colds, rashes, et cetera. Ask your Etheric Body if these symptoms are part of detoxification. (See discussion of Detoxification in Chapter VII.)

As a precautionary measure against any potential infections, viral or bacterial, which may invade the body during the period of a weakened immune system, it is wise to ask the Etheric Body on a daily basis to destroy the viruses and bacteria at the Etheric level. This procedure can help prevent any new infections from attacking the Physical Body.

As this disease focuses its attack on the body's immune system, it is particularly advisable to call upon a spiritual healing source which is especially effective in strengthening the immune system This spirit source is known as The White Healing Light. (See Chapter V under Other Energy Sources.)

Proper nutrition, including nutritional supplements are essential to help restore the health of the immune system. Immune system enhancers are products designed for this purpose and are available at most health food stores.

Regarding medical testing, the standard tests currently used for "T" cells and immune system deficiency do *not* tell you whether the HIV virus is out of the body or not. It takes a very long time for the immune system and the "T" cells to recover, even after the virus is out of the body.

As of the end of 1996, only a test for the HIV virus itself, or the Burden Viral Load test gave you a more accurate assessment.

In doing Bio-Etheric Healing, after you have asked the Deva to get the HIV virus out of the body, you can assess the progress of this work and also, if and when it has been completed. Just ask the Etheric Body from time to time regarding the status of the work.

When the Etheric Body tells you that the HIV virus is out of the body completely, you should ask it if the drugs you have been using are to be continued or stopped. If the Etheric Body wants you to continue, ask it for how long, specifying time periods such as a week, or a month, etc., so as to make it easier for the Etheric Body to respond. After that time has elapsed, ask the Etheric Body again about the need for drugs. The goal here is to get off the drugs as soon as possible because these drugs are usually strong and can harm your body by attacking healthy cells.

When asking the Etheric Body if any of the drugs being taken are needed any longer, you must do this by holding each drug, individually, in the hand. Then, using one's Communication Skills, ask the Etheric Body whether the drug is still needed. Repeat on a daily basis for those drugs still needed. You might ask also if the drug is needed in smaller doses or every other day before stopping it altogether.

HYPOGLYCEMIA

Hypoglycemia involves the Solar Plexus Chakra (#3) and the Third Eye Chakra (#6). It may be treated by healing the pancreas via the chakras. Ask the Etheric Body which chakra(s) and vortices are involved. Ask the Etheric Body to break up any blocked energy, to balance and to clear the chakra(s) and vortices involved. Also, ask the Etheric Body to heal the pancreas. This process will take an extended period of time for results. Keep checking the Etheric Body and repeat process as needed.

IMPOTENCE

Impotence may involve the Sacral Chakra (#2). Ask the Etheric Body to tell you if this chakra or its vortices are blocked, cloudy, unbalanced, or damaged. Ask the Etheric Body to clear, repair, balance, or remove blocked energy of the Sacral Chakra and its vortices, whichever is needed. Please ask for one procedure to be worked on at a time. Repeat as necessary.

INCONTINENCE

Ask the Etheric Body to strengthen the bladder. It may do so.

INDIGESTION

Indigestion may be a complex problem because of the wide variety of causes or their combination. Also, each individual attack may be the result of a different cause and not related to a previous attack. However, it is most likely that indigestion relates to a person's pattern and habits of food consumption and thus some study of one's behavior in this area can be very useful to approach the problem.

Essentially, indigestion involves the kind and amount of food we consume, and the ability of our body to process that food and make it available for the proper functioning of our body. In addition to the problems created by our lifestyle patterns in this regard, the general health of the stomach and digestive process is also subject to the condition of the Solar Plexus Chakra (#3), and the Throat Chakra (#5).

Ask your Etheric Body to help you determine the factor or factors contributing to your indigestion by reviewing the following possibilities with it and then take the appropriate action.

1. If your body doesn't have enough gastric fluid to digest the food, you can ask the Etheric Body to produce more digestive fluid, in the amount needed.

2. If this inadequacy of gastric fluid is a frequent occurrence, you may need to use supplements, such as betaine hydrochloride tablets after meals, but only after obtaining your Physical Body's permission. Do not take these acid supplements if there is any ulcer problem. (In the case of recurring

indigestion or too much acid, please consult your medical professional.)

3. In the case of indigestion related to a blocked or cloudy chakra, ask your Etheric Body to determine if the Solar Plexus Chakra, or the Throat Chakra, or both, are involved. Once the problem is identified, ask the Etheric Body to break up blocked energy and/or to clear the cloudiness of the chakra and vortices involved.

4. In the case of occasional indigestion, gas pain, or bloating, you may need to review your eating habits. Avoid eating too much at one time, or avoid eating more white flour products and sugars than your body can handle. A change of diet to keep your acid-alkali ratio at normal levels is in order. A more acid than alkali level in the body is deemed important for better health. (See section on Nutrition in Chapter VII.) It is also wise to avoid drinking too much water or other liquids while eating, because this tends to dilute the body's digestive juices at a time when they are needed.

5. Check your Etheric Body to see if you have an allergic reaction to some foods, or the spices used in their preparation. If so, stop eating them or avoid them as much as possible.

6. In some cases of continuing indigestion, the problem may be caused by parasites which have come into the digestive system via food or drink. (See separate section under Intestinal Parasites/Parasites.)

7. Lastly, if your indigestion is due to eating spoiled or contaminated food, see your medical professional.

INFECTIONS (GENERAL)

At the first sign of an infection, tell the Etheric Body to knock out and destroy all viruses and bacteria that have come into the body and are causing the infection.

When a person is in a situation where he or she is in contact with many people, it is good caution to use protective measures. Every morning (or night), ask the Etheric Body to destroy any viral or bacterial infections that might enter the body and do it harm. Repeat as necessary.

For additional help, you may provide your body with nutritional support. Take one-half or a full gram of vitamin C and 500 milligrams of chelated zinc once or twice a day.

INFECTIOUS HEPATITIS

This disease is an acute inflammation of the liver caused by a virus. It is often characterized by fever, nausea, vomiting, abdominal pain and jaundice. In its active stage, this disease is highly contagious. A major result of this disease is liver damage. Also, the virus itself stays in the body so that the disease is transmittable to others in blood transfusions.

Infectious hepatitis may also involve the Solar Plexus Chakra (#3) causing underactivity and sometimes blockages in energy flow. Ask the Etheric Body to help by removing any traces of the infectious hepatitis virus out of the Physical Body, and also, out of the bloodstream. Then ask the Etheric Body, in separate requests, to unblock and balance the Solar Plexus Chakra and its vortices.

After this, ask the Etheric Body to remove the Miasm of infectious hepatitis from the Base Chakra (#1) of the Etheric Body. Finally, ask the Etheric Body to heal any damage to the liver. This entire procedure should be repeated as often as necessary until communication with the Etheric Body tells you that the virus is out of the body and there is a total recovery.

Sometimes Karma can be a factor in some cases of this disease. Check your Etheric Body to see if Karma is involved. If it is, see separate section on Karma in this chapter for further instruction.

Even if you have had this disease a long time ago, the virus would still be in the Physical Body because that is its nature. Therefore, the same procedures offered above should be followed in this case, and removal of the virus would be possible.

INFERTILITY
(Channeled by Kwan Yin)

Infertility in both men and women may involve the Sacral Chakra (#2). Ask the Etheric Body if this chakra or its vortices are blocked or cloudy. If there is blockage, ask the Etheric Body to unblock the chakra or its vortices, as appropriate. If the problem is cloudiness, ask the Etheric Body to clear the chakra and its vortices, as needed.

INTESTINAL PARASITES/PARASITES
(Channeled by Kwan Yin)

References to parasites in the body are almost always thought of as being intestinal parasites. However, parasites could also reside in other parts of the body, for example, the spleen, the bladder, etc.

Using Bio-Etheric Healing, it is now possible to get parasites, wherever they reside, out of the body, effectively without drugs. This would also include tapeworm and other parasites. To do so, ask the Etheric Body to clear these parasites out of the Physical Body, wherever they reside.

However, please be mindful that as this occurs, detoxification will result. A person needs to drink a lot of water to help the detoxification process.

KARMA RELATED TO ILLNESS
(Channeled by Edgar Cayce)

Less recognized than any other cause of ill health, Karma is of vital importance in the life of an individual. No one is free from its effects, and the effects of Karma can lead to good health and good luck, or conversely to poor health and bad luck. When working with healing energies, as in Bio-Etheric Healing, you have the power to clear the Karma of someone who is ill, and start that person on the road to wellness. If Karma is involved in an illness, it must be addressed first and removed first, as it overrides any directions to the Etheric Body for healing.

However, a major exception to this rule comes into play when the illness is caused by bacteria or viruses and, at the same time, Karma is found to be involved. In such situations, the bacteria or viruses must be removed *first,* as they are of more immediate danger by causing the illness to progress in the body. Also it may be that the illness requires immediate medical attention. Therefore, the removal of the Karma which takes more time and which serves to prevent future occurrences of the illness, can await recovery.

Karma resides in the two outer layers of the Aura, the ones not visible or named. Karma can interfere with the normal functioning of the Physical Body and its immune system, and affect the Emotional Body as well. It can interfere with recovery from illness, whereby one cannot seem to shake off one illness after another, without any apparent explanation. That is Karma at work. With

Bio-Etheric Healing you can ask your Etheric Body if Karma is a factor in your illness. If the answer is positive, ask your Etheric Body to erase the Karma involved in your illness from your Aura. Illnesses as a result of an HIV positive condition are not subject to Karmic influence.

KARMA RELATED TO LUCK

In a sense, Karma is the cumulative effect of one's deeds, thoughts, and actions over many lifetimes. It is the result of the past, and its action can affect the present and the future of one's life.

Karma plays a role in the way the scenario of one's life is played out, and can be the cause of success or failure in our present life relating to business or personal relationships.

If you wish to know about a specific situation that is working out negatively for you (in business or personal relationships), ask your Etheric Body if Karma has any relevance to the situation. If the answer is "yes," and you want to change the course of the way things are going, this is what you do. Tell your Etheric Body to get rid of or destroy the bad Karma that is causing you the problem in this specific situation. Ask it to remove the bad Karma from the outer two layers of the Aura, where it resides. Give it two weeks to a month. If the Karma is very thick, it may take longer.

KIDNEY PROBLEMS

Malfunction of the Base Chakra (#1) may be involved in kidney problems. Use your Communication Skills to find out if it is relevant. Check the Base Chakra and its vortices to see if they are cloudy, damaged, or blocked. Then ask the Etheric Body to heal, clear, and/or unblock the chakra and vortices, as needed.

LARYNGITIS

Laryngitis involves the Throat Chakra (#5). Ask the Etheric Body to clear or break up any blocked energy that may be involved in the laryngitis.

LIVER PROBLEMS

Liver problems may involve the Solar Plexus Chakra (#3). Check to see if the problem is related to a cloudy, blocked, out-of-balance, or damaged chakra. Then ask the Etheric Body to clear, repair, or remove the blocked energy or balance this chakra, accordingly. Repeat as needed. Also, ask the Etheric Body to heal the liver and bring it up to normal functioning.

For liver damage resulting from hepatitis, see Infectious Hepatitis.

LUPUS

(Channeled by Kwan Yin)

This disease is caused by an organism which is under the jurisdiction of the Devic Kingdom, governed by Pan. Therefore, in treating both Lupus Discoid and Lupus Erythematosus, it is necessary to use your Communication Skills to ask to speak to the Deva of the specific organism involved. Once contact has been established, ask the Deva involved to get the organism of that disease out of the body.

Lupus Discoid

Lupus may cause a the dysfunction of the immune system. Ask the Etheric Body to heal the immune system where it is malfunctioning. Then ask it to correct the imbalance of the Heart Chakra (#4) and its vortices and to clear the blockage and cloudiness of the chakra.

Lupus Erythematosus

This a very complex illness with many components possible, all of which need to be investigated.

One component may be related to a dysfunction of the immune system. Ask the Etheric Body to correct the dysfunction of the immune system that is causing lupus erythematosus.

Another component may be a problem within the Chakra System. There may be more than one chakra involved. The Heart Chakra (#4) is always involved. Check the entire chakra field to see which chakra(s) or vortice(s) are malfunctioning and what is causing the malfunction. Check each to see whether it requires balancing, clearing, unblocking, or repairing damage. Ask the Etheric

Body to heal each accordingly, addressing each chakra and its vortices individually. Make sure the entire chakra field is brought up to maximum functioning, that is, balanced, repaired, unblocked, and cleared.

Other possible components may be anxiety or fear, or Traumas or Karma of past lives, or Traumas of present life. Ask the Etheric Body to tell you which of these possibilities, if any, are involved. (See sections on Anxiety/Fear, Traumas and Karma.)

If Traumas are involved, get permission from the Soul before asking the Etheric Body to remove the related Trauma from the Aura.

If Karma is implicated, ask the Etheric Body to get the Karma from past lives causing this problem to be removed from the two outer layers of the Aura.

Another possible component of this illness may be psychological. Check the Etheric Body to see if there is a psychological component in this case. If so, professional psychological help should be sought.

For any damage to the Physical Body caused by this disease, ask the Etheric Body to heal the damage, using the Ketheric Template (7th layer of the Aura) as a blueprint of a healthy body to indicate the repair needed. This request needs to be repeated for better results.

As this complex disease requires much work with the Etheric Body, be sure to space your requests so as not to overload it.

During this time of treatment and healing, consume only those foods providing maximum nutrition to aid the body in its effort to repair itself. Use no white flour or sugar in any form in the diet. A diet high in protein and potassium should be maintained. Use a strong vitamin and mineral formula, vitamin E (400 IU's), stress formula (vitamins B and C), as well as any commercial version of a Pep Power formula sold in health food stores.

LYME DISEASE

Lyme disease is in the syphilis family. It is a complex disease and requires several different procedures to help dispel it and treat the damage it causes. It must be caught early to provide a chance for better results and the possible avoidance of its most debilitating effects. At the first sign of infection, ask the Etheric Body to remove the infection from the body. Then ask the Etheric Body to remove the Miasm for Lyme disease from the Base Chakra (#1), where it resides.

If the disease was not caught early and physical damage occurs, ask the Etheric Body to repair the physical damage. Ask it to do so by using the Ketheric Template (7th layer of the Aura) to provide a blueprint of the healthy body, thus revealing the damaged areas requiring structural repairs. Then, ask the Etheric Body to break up pain by releasing blocked energy. Do this as necessary, being careful to name the specific location of the pain.

Lyme disease leaves bacteria called spirochetes in the body which reside in the soft tissue and cannot be reached by antibiotics. They can reactivate the disease at any time and, therefore, it is critical to rid the body of them. With Bio-Etheric Healing, the spirochetes are naturally removed from their hiding places by the Etheric Body.

If you have had Lyme disease in the past that was successfully treated by antibiotics, it is quite likely that some spirochetes still remain in the soft tissue of your body. As a precaution against their ability to reactivate the disease, it is wise to ask the Etheric Body to remove them from the Physical Body.

(Originally, I had worked with the Deva of the deer tick to heal Lyme disease. Subsequently, I've found that working with the Etheric Body directly is faster and more efficient in getting spirochetes out of the body completely.)

MENSTRUAL IRREGULARITIES

Menstrual irregularities may be related to the Throat Chakra (#5). Problems may arise due to imbalance of this chakra or its vortices. Ask the Etheric Body to balance this chakra and its vortices. For pain, ask the Etheric Body to break up any blocked energy.

Menstrual problems may also be caused by an insufficiency of specific vitamins and minerals in the diet; namely, calcium/magnesium, vitamin B-6, B-complex, or vitamin E. For each of these, ask the Etheric Body if there is an insufficiency. Where an insufficiency exists, plan to supplement your diet with the necessary vitamins or minerals in their recommended daily dosages.

METAL POISONING

(Channeled by Kwan Yin)

Chelation therapy for removing metal poisoning may be possible by using Bio-Etheric Healing. This should be accomplished by asking the Etheric Body to combine the specific metal particles involved with protein particles (which abound in the body) and to remove them from the Physical Body via the normal channels. This process of combining elements is called chelation. Protein particles are available for this chelation process for metal particle removal as the body itself is primarily protein, and in the normal process of cell regeneration, protein cells get separated.

There are many different kinds of protein particles for the metal to bond with. The bonding occurs because there is an affinity between metals and the protein particles. It is a chemical reaction. Yet, unless the Etheric Body is asked to pair the specific metal causing the metal poisoning, it will not do so on its own. The offending metals which work best with this chelation procedure are aluminum, lead, mercury, and cadmium.

This procedure does have a detoxification period for the poisoning to leave the body. In fact, the whole chelation therapy process is to detoxify the body from the toxic effects of the metal. These toxic effects can be quite severe and so, the detoxification itself may be long and difficult. If you ask your Etheric Body to ease the discomfort of detoxification, it will do so.

MIASMS

(Channeled by Kwan Yin)

Strictly speaking, a Miasm is not a disease. It is a predisposition to a specific disease and, as such, represents a major factor in illness. Miasms reside in the Base Chakra (#1). Removing the Miasm for a particular disease can be extremely effective (possibly 70%) in preventing that disease from occurring or returning. Miasms can be inherited; they can be picked up by the Etheric Body from the air; they can be the result of earlier diseases, or such things as toxins (both chemical and viral), x-rays, radiation, et cetera. It appears that almost all diseases have Miasms, including cancer, syphilis, TB, Alzheimer's disease, colitis, shingles, and diphtheria. Check your own family history and ask your own Etheric Body to indicate which Miasms of which illnesses exist in your Base Chakra, asking about each illness individually.

It is important in treating a particular disease, to ask the Etheric Body to remove the Miasm for that disease from the Base Chakra. You may feel tired while this clearing out is taking place, and you may experience other symptoms of detoxification as well. Work on only one Miasm at a time so you do not overload the system. Where no disease is present but a Miasm for it exists, it is wise as a preventative measure to remove the Miasm from the Base Chakra.

MIGRAINE HEADACHES
(Channeled by Kwan Yin)

The basic cause of migraine headaches is an imbalance of the two sides of the brain. To rectify this, ask the Etheric Body to bring the two sides of the brain back into proper balance. To guide the Etheric Body in the process, tell it to use the Ketheric Template (7th layer of the Aura) as a model as to where the balance needs to be corrected. This request should be repeated monthly until healing takes place.

As the Brain itself is a major player in Bio-Etheric Healing (see discussion on the role of the Brain in Chapter II), it is advisable to ask it for its cooperation in this balancing and healing procedure. It is important to ask each side of the brain, separately addressed as "the left side" and "the right side" for this cooperation to ensure better results.

Migraines also may be related to the Alta Major Chakra, which may be blocked or cloudy. Ask the Etheric Body to break up blocked energy of the Alta Major Chakra and vortices that may be causing the pain. Also ask the Etheric Body to clear the chakra, if necessary.

MULTIPLE SCLEROSIS
(Channeled by Kwan Yin)

It may be possible to use Bio-Etheric Healing in work with multiple sclerosis. As difficult a challenge as this disease may pose, this logic derives from the fact that the disease is caused by an as yet unidentified organism. Therefore, the organism for it must be under the jurisdiction of the Devic Kingdom, with its leader, Pan (see Chapter VI). However, before the actual healing steps are taken, it is wise to ask if Karma is involved. If so, Karma related to this disease must be removed from the outer two layers of the Aura. (See listing under Karma.)

A first step in the healing process is to ask for the Deva of the multiple sclerosis organism. Upon successful contact, ask that Deva to get the organism out of the body. You may have to make contact with the Deva, perhaps monthly, to check on what progress is being made in ridding the body of this organism and repeat the request if necessary.

However, be prepared for a difficult detoxification process which may also be drawn out. Review the discussion of detoxification in Chapter VII and follow the procedures indicated to ease this process.

At the same time, a characteristic of this disease is its deteriorating effect on the nerves and throughout the body causing further harm. Ask the Etheric Body to restore to their normal condition, the outside layers of nerves that have become afflicted. Ask the Etheric Body to do this by using the Ketheric Template (7th layer of the Aura) as a blueprint to what healthy outside layers of nerves should be like. Also ask the Etheric Body to create the chemicals needed to strengthen the outer layer of the nerves so they no longer disintegrate. It is a lack of these chemicals which protect the nerve fibers from attack by free radical oxidants in the body that leads to the destruction of nerve tissue throughout the body. This request should be repeated twice a month for best results. (See section on Free Radical Oxidants.)

In addition, it is important to ask the Etheric Body to remove the free radical oxidants from within the Physical Body. Make this request at regular intervals, at least once a month.

MYASTHENIA GRAVIS
(Channeled by Kwan Yin)

This is a disease of the voluntary muscles which is characterized by a progressive weakness without any atrophy or sensory disturbance. There is loss of control of these muscles. This disease is believed to be one of the auto-immune diseases and, therefore, one of its triggers may involve the body's reaction to an unidentified fear.

Myasthenia gravis involves the Heart Chakra (#4), which becomes blocked as a result of this unidentified fear. Ask the

Etheric Body to unblock the energy in the Heart Chakra and its vortices. Also ask the Etheric Body to balance the Heart Chakra and its vortices.

It is wise to follow the same suggestions provided for other fear-related problems. (See Anxiety/Fear, Trauma, and Karma.)

NECK PAIN AND STIFFNESS

Pain and stiffness in the neck may be affected by blockage of the Throat Chakra (#5) and its vortices. The Alta Major Chakra may also be blocked. Ask the Etheric Body for each chakra individually, if it is involved. For the chakra(s) implicated ask the Etheric Body to break up any blocked energy and to clear the chakra and vortices as needed. Sometimes neck pain and stiffness is caused by remnants of past life Traumas or Karma. Refer to sections on Karma and Traumas if your Etheric Body determines that to be the case.

NEURALGIA

(Channeled by Kwan Yin)

Neuralgia may be due to blocked energy. If the neuralgia is located on the right side, it may involve the Third Eye Chakra (#6); if it is located on the left side, it may involve the Throat Chakra (#5). Ask the Etheric Body to break up any blockage in these chakras and then to clear them and their vortices of any cloudiness.

NEUROMA

Neuromas are very painful growths attached to the nerves in the ball of the feet. Surgical removal of this growth may result in nerve damage or loss. Moreover, surgery does not always have a high chance of success, and the possibility of the neuroma returning is always there. Bio-Etheric Healing offers the possibility for a slow shrinking of the neuroma and separating the neuroma from the nerve itself, leaving the nerve intact. This treatment involves removal of the neuroma at the Etheric Level which, in turn, should lead to a slow shrinking of the neuroma at the Physical Level, because its roots in the Aura are gone.

Ask the Etheric Body to make room for the removal of the neuroma at the Etheric Template (the 5th layer of the Aura which is in negative space). Then ask the Etheric Body to use the Ketheric

Template (7th layer of the Aura) as a blueprint to what a healthy foot should be. Then ask the Etheric Body to remove the neuroma from the Aura at the Etheric Level.

Ask the Etheric Body to have the Physical Body separate the neuroma from the nerve in the foot, and then ask it to shrink or dissolve it out of the body as well. If there is pain involved, ask the Etheric Body to remove the blocked energy causing that pain, specifying the location of the pain. This is a very safe but slow process, and needs to be repeated at intervals for greater progress.

As a means of hastening this very slow healing process, one might consider calling upon the energy of the spirit source known as The White Healing Light. (See Chapter V under Other Energy Sources.)

OBSESSIVE BEHAVIOR
Ask the Etheric Body to clear obsessive behavior from the Mental Body.

OSTEOARTHRITIS
Megavitamin therapy is recommended, using a strong multivitamin/mineral formula, including vitamins A, D, C, and E, and a careful diet is of prime importance in treating osteoarthritis. It is important to use sugar-free products and no white flour products. Then supplement with calcium and magnesium of the elemental and chelated kind (2,000 cal/1,000 mag) to start, tapering down when the body is greatly improved. The body must have acids to absorb calcium. Use cider vinegar in tabs or use cider vinegar mixed with oil (to protect the teeth enamel), in salad. It is also useful to use betaine hydrochloride in tabs (if there is no difficulty with ulcers) for absorption of the calcium/magnesium.

Ask the Etheric Body to heal the body of arthritis as quickly as possible and to use the Ketheric Template (7th layer of the Aura) as a guide. For pain, specify the area and ask the Etheric Body to break up any blocked energy causing the pain. Do this as often as necessary.

Ask the Etheric Body to produce collagen in the body, as needed, to repair any damaged connective tissue and to produce hyaluronic acid in the amounts needed to lubricate joints.

PAIN (GENERAL)

Much of the pain the body experiences may be due to blocked energy. Use your Communication Skills to verify if this is the case with any pain you are experiencing. It is important to do so because pain not due to blocked energy may be an indication of something more serious, and should be discussed with your medical professional. With blocked energy pain, ask your Etheric Body to remove the blockage, specifying the particular area either verbally or by placing your hand where the pain is located. The pain should soon dissipate. Repeat as often as necessary.

When there is pain of no known origin, it may be due to a Karmic situation or past life Traumas. If you get a positive response to either of these possibilities, you can ask the Etheric Body to search out which Traumas specifically are linked to that particular area of pain, and to remove all the past life Traumas involved. To do this you must first ask permission from the Soul. (See listing under Traumas.)

If Karma is causing the pain, ask the Etheric Body to locate the area of the Karma involved in that particular pain, and remove it from the two outer layers of the Aura. (See listing under Karma Related to Illness.)

For specific cases where pain is expected as part of a known process, such as dental work, childbirth, or overexertion, you can ask the Etheric Body to produce endorphins, in advance, as a possible aid to counteract the expected pain.

POISON IVY

When the first pustules appear, ask your Etheric Body to dry them up and keep any new ones from coming out. Ask your Etheric Body to remove the poison ivy completely out of your system. Then ask the Etheric Body to get the Miasm of poison ivy out of the Base Chakra (#1).

RHEUMATOID ARTHRITIS

Rheumatoid arthritis is one of a group of diseases characterized by pain and inflammation of the body's joints. In the long term, it can lead to persistent pain, stiffness and even deformity.

Karma may also be implicated in this disease. Ask the Etheric Body for confirmation. If Karma is involved, ask the Etheric Body to remove the Karma pertaining to this disease from the outer layers of the Aura as a first step. (See listing under Karma.)

Rheumatoid arthritis is caused by an organism which may be possible to remove by Bio-Etheric Healing. To do this one must first ask for the Deva of the rheumatoid arthritis organism, and upon contact, ask the Deva to get the organism out of the body. It may be wise to call upon the Deva several times over a three month period and ask her to remove the organism in stages so as to make this procedure less painful to endure.

As this disease is complicated and can affect many parts of the body over an extended period of time, there will probably be a difficult period of detoxification. See Chapter VII on Detoxification and review the discussion of procedures to help ease the process.

With this disease, the immune system is always involved. At the same time, anxiety and fear are implicated in rheumatoid arthritis, as with all other auto-immune diseases. Therefore, it is important to address both the healing of the auto-immune system and also the anxiety and fear.

Ask the Etheric Body to heal the immune system where it is malfunctioning. As for the fear and anxiety, these may present a more complex situation and it may be wise to seek the advice of a medical professional with psychological training. At the same time, as fear and anxiety always cause blockage of the Heart Chakra (#4), it is important to clear and unblock the Heart Chakra and to do this often over the period of time that the fear and anxiety persists. To do this, ask the Etheric Body to restore the proper functioning of the Heart Chakra and its vortices by clearing them and breaking up any blockages.

Sometimes when the fear is insidious and difficult to identify, it may be due to past life Traumas or present life Traumas. Ask the Etheric Body if this is the case, and if so, ask the Etheric Body to remove the Traumas from the Mental Body of the Aura. However, before doing this, you must first get the permission of the Soul. If the Soul does not agree to this, do not do it as there may be other important purposes served by the Trauma in protecting the body from other dangers in its present life.

A further step is to ask the Etheric Body to remove the Miasm of the disease out of the Base Chakra (#1) to help prevent future attacks.

For pain, ask the Etheric Body to remove blocked energy from the specific area involved. When inflammation is involved, it may indicate a blocked or cloudy chakra or vortices in the inflamed area. Ask the Etheric Body to unblock and/or clear the chakra(s) that is affecting the area inflamed. Ask the Etheric Body to release all unnecessary fluids from the joints via the normal channels.

Bio-Etheric Healing may be helpful in another way with rheumatoid arthritis. A common inflammatory protein which is usually found in this disease is TNF-alpha or tumor necrosis factor alpha. This protein can set off a chemical action which involves inflammation and damage to joints. TNF-alpha is one of a group of substances known as cytokines which are found in people with this disease. The direction of recent medical treatment is to find and use drugs that can block the action of TNF-alpha and other cytokines. With Bio-Etheric Healing, it may be possible to stop the destructive action of cytokines by removing them from the body. Ask the Etheric Body to remove any destructive cytokines, particularly the TNF-alpha protein, from the Physical Body.

As a means of helping the body to recover from some of the damage from this disease and to restore it to more normal flexibility and health, here are some additional suggestions:

- Ask the Etheric Body to enlist the aid of the Physical Body to produce collagen (connective tissue) to repair joints where collagen is damaged.
- For the typical growths, nodules, and bumps which result from rheumatoid arthritis, ask the Etheric Body to remove them by first making room for them in the Etheric Template (the 5th layer of the Aura, which is a negative space template). Then ask the Etheric Body to remove the growths by using the Ketheric Template (7th layer of the Aura) as a blueprint of what a healthy body looks like.
- Ask the Etheric Body to heal affected joints, making them more flexible and returning them to normal, again using the Ketheric Template as a guide.
- Ask the Physical Body to produce hyaluronic acid as a lubricant for the joints.

Repeat these requests as often as necessary.

- During the healing process, which may be extensive, use any additional therapeutic procedures such as exercise, Massage Therapy, Therapeutic Touch, Reiki, et cetera, whichever will give you the most comfort while you are in need.
- Vitamin and mineral supplements and a proper diet is essential to aid in the healing process. Do not use sugar or white flour products. Use cider vinegar in salad dressings or take cider vinegar pills or betaine hydrochloride supplements as needed to absorb calcium. Take 2,000-3,500 mg of calcium (elemental and chelated) with one-half of that amount of magnesium (in tablets that have both). Also take a multi-vitamin that contains C, D, A and E to absorb the calcium. Include a strong multimineral as well. Take additional vitamin C in doses applicable to your body's needs. Take ginger capsules (or ginger powder) twice per day. Check the vitamin dosages needed regularly by using Communication Skills to see how much of each vitamin your body requires. As you become well, your body will require less of everything.

One caution to note is that in the case of ulcers, do not take additional acid in any form without first asking your medical professional.

(Also see separate listing under Bone Related Problems.)

SCIATICA
(Channeled by Kwan Yin)

Sciatica may involve one or more of three chakras, namely, the Base Chakra (#1), the Sacral Chakra (#2), or the Solar Plexus Chakra (#3). It may be involved with the blockage of energy in these chakras or their vortices. Using your Communication Skills, you need to find out if any of these chakras are involved and which one(s). For each chakra involved, you must ask the Etheric Body to unblock the energy of that chakra and its vortices. Repeat this procedure as needed. If you are not able to ascertain which chakras are involved, simply ask the Etheric Body to break up any blocked energy that is causing the pain. Name the area of pain, or show where the pain is with your hand placement. Again, repeat as often as needed.

SHINGLES

Shingles is caused by a virus that is in the chickenpox family. Ask the Etheric Body to remove the viral infection from the body. Ask the Etheric Body to dry up the pustules. Ask the Etheric Body to prevent additional pustules from erupting on the skin. Ask the Etheric Body to remove blocked energy that is causing pain.

The nervous system is involved in shingles, and the pain and pustules generally follow the meridian of the nerve. Acupuncture has been found to be effective here because the treatment itself works directly on the nerves involved, following the meridian.

In the case where acupuncture is not available, or not of interest, Bio-Etheric Healing may offer relief. There are several chakras that may be involved; namely, the Base Chakra, the Solar Plexus Chakra (#3), the Third Eye Chakra (#6), and the Crown Chakra (#7). Ask the Etheric Body specifically for each chakra and its vortices to confirm which chakra(s) and vortices are involved. For each one involved, ask the Etheric Body if it is blocked or cloudy. Then ask the Etheric Body to unblock and/or clear the chakra and vortices involved. Finally, ask the Etheric Body to remove the Miasm for shingles from the Base Chakra (#1) to help in the prevention of future attacks.

SINUS

Sinus problems involve blockage or cloudiness of the Third Eye Chakra (#6). Ask the Etheric Body to clear this chakra and remove any blocked energy from the chakra and its vortices. Repeat as necessary.

SKIN PROBLEMS

Skin Eruptions

Skin eruptions may involve the Solar Plexus Chakra (#3), the Third Eye Chakra (#6), the Throat Chakra (#5), and the Base Chakra (#1), or their vortices. The involvement is an overactivity of one or more of these chakras. Ask the Etheric Body which of these chakras and their vortices are involved. Then ask the Etheric Body to balance the activity of the chakra or chakras and their vortices which are involved.

Wrinkles, Dry Skin, Blemishes

These skin problems may involve blockage of the Third Eye Chakra (#6) or the Throat Chakra (#5) and their vortices. Ask the Etheric Body which chakra(s) is involved and blocked. Ask the Etheric Body to break up the blocked energy in the chakra(s) implicated. In the case with wrinkles, this request will need to be made on a regularly scheduled basis.

SLEEP DISORDERS

Sleep disorders can have many causes that may be difficult to pinpoint. Also, they can result from a combination of factors. Some of the factors involved include a malfunction of the Crown Chakra (#7) and/or the Third Eye Chakra (#6), a disorder of the brain cells, obsessive behavior, restless-leg syndrome, fear that may go back to early childhood Traumas, or past-life Traumas, Karma, continuous brain activity that doesn't allow one to sleep, nutritional deficiencies, and possibly other factors that are unique to the individual.

Start by asking your Etheric Body about each of these potential causes, individually, to see which one or ones are involved in your case. Then, for each of the factors you find is involved, here is the suggested remedial action to take:

- Ask the Etheric Body of the person if the Crown Chakra (#7) and the Third Eye Chakra (#6) are involved. Then ask if each of the chakras are blocked, damaged, cloudy, or unbalanced. To treat, ask the Etheric Body to break up the blockage, clear the cloudiness, repair the damage, or balance the chakra involved. It is also a good idea to check the whole chakra field. When asking the Etheric Body to work with the chakras, please request one function for one chakra at a time, so as not to overload the system.
- Restless-leg syndrome is a twitchy, wormy feeling in the legs or feet which causes much tossing and turning, thus interfering with sleep. If this problem is confirmed by the Etheric Body, ask it to calm the Physical Body, especially concentrating on the lower body. Make this request each night at bedtime. In some cases, this restless-leg problem may be the result of a deficiency of the B-complex vitamin. Supplementing the diet with this vitamin in a tablet form would also be very

helpful. It may be that a disorder of the brain cells governing the legs is implicated. If so, ask the Etheric Body to repair this dysfunction by using the Ketheric Template (7th layer of the Aura) as a blueprint of what the healthy brain cells which govern the legs should be. Repeat this request daily until cells are repaired.

- If the problem is one of fear, Traumas, or Karma, please refer to the appropriate section on Karma, Anxiety/Fear or Trauma.
- If the problem is one of continuous brain activity, ask the Etheric Body to clear the Mental Body each night at bedtime.
- The Mental Body is also involved in obsessive behavior (such as continuous repetition of a thought, a song, et cetera) that interferes with sleep. In this case, ask the Etheric Body to get the obsessive behavior out of the Mental Body and to calm the Mental Body.
- A nutritional deficiency of other needed ingredients for a healthy functioning of the body may be causing interference with proper sleep. You can check your Etheric Body for some of these to see what may be the lack. Sometimes, with a fat-free diet, the body may develop a dry, itchy skin because it is not getting the proper amount of fatty acids or oils required to process the oil-related vitamins it gets in the food it consumes. Be sure to consume the equivalent of two tablespoons of oil a day. Canola or any other cooking oil could be taken.

SORE THROAT

For a sore throat due to a viral or bacterial infection, ask the Etheric Body to destroy the virus or bacteria causing the problem. Sore throats may involve blocked energy of the Throat Chakra (#5) or cloudiness, or even damage to this chakra. Ask the Etheric Body which of these three potential problems exist and then ask the Etheric Body to treat accordingly, that is, either breaking up the blocked energy, clearing, or repairing this chakra and its vortices.

With sore throats or hoarseness that doesn't go away, there may be other reasons, some of them serious, and this situation needs to be brought to the attention of your medical doctor.

SPASTIC COLON
(Channeled by Kwan Yin)

This is primarily a stress-related problem. Anxiety and fear caused by Traumas of current or past lives may create blockages of the Heart Chakra (#4) or its vortices. Meditation is recommended to relieve present stress. Also, you should ask the Etheric Body to release Traumas of present and past lives from the Mental Body of the Aura. However, before doing this, you must first get approval from the Soul to do so, using your Communication Skills. Do not do so if the Soul does not grant permission because it is likely that these Traumas may be serving a useful purpose protecting you from a greater or more real threat to your present life.

Ask the Etheric Body to break up any blocked energy in the Heart Chakra or its vortices and to clear up any cloudiness there. As anger is often a component of this problem, ask the Etheric Body to clear and release anger from the Emotional Body. Be sure to make these requests in stages, say, at one week intervals to give the Physical Body time to adjust and recover.

Finally, to relieve any immediate anxiety, ask the Etheric Body to clear the Emotional Body and do this as needed. In the case of immediate anxiety, it would be useful to first meditate and get calm and centered before communicating with your Etheric Body. (See also sections on Anxiety/Fear and Trauma.)

SPINAL PROBLEMS
Scoliosis (Curvature of the Spine)
(Channeled by Kwan Yin)

Scoliosis is a condition in which there develops a lateral curvature of the spine. To help in the healing, you must first ask the Etheric Body to begin straightening the spine by using the Ketheric Template (the 7th layer of the Aura) as a guide to what the normal position of the spine should be. Depending on the severity of the problem, this procedure may take a long time. Be patient. Over this period, it is wise to repeat this request and to check on the progress.

Scoliosis may be related to dysfunction of the Base Chakra (#1) and the Alta Major Chakra, and their vortices. Dietary problems may also be implicated. For example, improper absorption or utilization of calcium and magnesium taken from food by the body, or the insufficiency of these minerals in the diet are possibilities.

It is necessary to identify if dietary problems and/or problems with proper functioning of the chakras are at play. First, ask your Etheric Body for each of these factors, individually, if it is involved. If chakras or their vortices are involved, ask the Etheric Body for each one (Base or Alta major) if it is blocked, cloudy or damaged. Then, ask the Etheric Body to unblock or clear or repair the appropriate chakra(s) and vortices, as needed. (Also see listing on "Bone Related Problems.")

If dietary problems are involved, ask your Etheric Body if your calcium and magnesium intake is sufficient and, separately, ask if the absorption of these essential minerals is adequate to deliver your body's requirements.

If your calcium or magnesium intake is insufficient, be sure to include more of the foods in your diet which can provide them or take a calcium/magnesium formula tablet supplement in a combination of two parts calcium to one part magnesium. It is best to find these in both chelated form (for better absorption) and elemental form (for more of the active ingredient).

If your intake of these minerals is sufficient, but your body's absorption of them is insufficient, ask your Etheric Body individually if the problem is a lack of sufficient digestive juices or if it is interference with the work of the digestive system caused by other factors such as too much sugar, or processed white flour products (such as bread, pastry, or pasta) in the diet. It is best to substitute whole grain flour products instead for their greater nutritive value.

If the problem is one of faulty absorption, it is wise to reduce the intake of sugars in all their forms (honey, syrups, fructose, sweets, et cetera). One may also need to add vinegar to the diet, or other forms of digestive aids, such as vinegar tablets or betaine hydrochloride tablets as needed. Use your Communication Skills to ask your Etheric Body what dosages are needed.

It is possible that the body's production of digestive juices is not adequate. If that is the case (confirm this with the Etheric Body), you may ask the Etheric Body to raise the level of the digestive juices to its normal level. Ask the Etheric body to do this using the Ketheric Template (7th layer of the Aura) as a guide to what the proper level of digestive juices should be for your body under normal conditions. This will only work well for you, however, if you remember that "normal" conditions means that you do not consume the sugars mentioned in the preceding paragraphs which throw off the body's normal acid/alkaline balance.

Injured/Ruptured Discs
(Channeled by Kwan Yin)

For injured or ruptured discs, ask the Etheric Body to use the Ketheric Template (7th layer of the Aura) as a blueprint of a healthy disc and to retrieve any lost cells and place them back into the injured or ruptured disc(s) within their outer layer. In addition, ask the Etheric Body to strengthen and repair this outer layer of the disc(s). Ask the Etheric Body to repair damaged cells or create new cells for the damaged disc(s) and to have them conform to the specifications for a healthy disc as revealed in the Ketheric Template.

As pain always accompanies such disc problems, ask the Etheric Body to break up the blocked energy causing the pain, mentioning the specific areas of pain. Repeat as needed.

Missing Discs

In the case of a disc missing due to complete deterioration, it may be possible to replace the missing disc. Ask the Etheric Body to replace the missing disc(s) by using the Ketheric Template (7th layer of the Aura) as a blueprint for what comprises a healthy disc and for the proper location of this new disc in the spine. Ask the Etheric Body to break up blocked energy to ease the pain caused by this problem, mentioning the specific site of the pain.

In all this work with the spine, expect any progress to take time, perhaps a year or more to replace a missing disc. Over this period, a reminder request for this work to the Etheric Body would be wise from time to time. However, as pain is often quite constant, more frequent requests for relief of pain, as often as needed, should be made of the Etheric Body.

STRESS

Stress is a mental tension resulting from current factors in a person's environment that tend to alter the normal peace or equilibrium. Extreme or continual or unrelieved stress may be a factor in disease causation. (See Anxiety/Fear and also Trauma sections.)

For simple stress encountered in the emotional situations of our daily lives, Bio-Etheric Healing may offer relief. Ask the Etheric Body to clear the Emotional Body. Repeat as needed.

STROKES
(Channeled by Ignatious)

Ignatious states that strokes often involve blocked energy in the Third Eye Chakra (#2) and its vortices. However, he cautions that his suggestions for remedy do not provide results which are certain.

First, ask the Etheric Body to break up the blocked energy in the Third Eye Chakra and its vortices and also to clear up any cloudiness there. Then, ask the Etheric Body to repair any damage to the brain caused by the stroke using the Ketheric Template (7th layer of the Aura) as a blueprint for what a healthy brain looks like. Ask the Etheric Body to ask the brain itself to help in this repair.

Finally, ask the Etheric Body to repair all the secondary damage caused elsewhere to the Physical Body, again using the Ketheric Template as a guide.

Repeat the entire procedure twice a day until progress is noted, before reducing this to once daily.

TEETH PROBLEMS (DUE TO BONE LOSS)

Bone loss in teeth can result from a variety of factors, including improper diet (such as too much sugars, not enough calcium, phosphorus, and vitamin D), improper absorption of calcium by the digestive system, pregnancy, and other stresses which result in emotional and chemical changes in the body, and also a lack of the important ingredient of collagen. Bone loss in the teeth, in turn, can lead to other teeth problems such as sensitivity and pain, tooth decay, and tooth loss.

Two factors critical to preventing bone loss, and helpful in its remedy are the adequacy of calcium (its intake, as well as absorption by the body) and collagen, the chief constituent of connective tissue and bones.

With Bio-Etheric Healing one may be able to get the Physical Body to produce the needed collagen in the amounts necessary for maintenance of healthy teeth, as well as for remedying bone loss. Therefore, in the case of tooth problems due to inadequate collagen, ask your Etheric body to have the Physical Body produce the collagen it needs in the required quantity to repair any bone loss in the mouth or teeth. Then, ask the Etheric Body to repair the bone loss using the Ketheric Template (7th layer of the Aura) as a blueprint of what a healthy mouth and/or teeth should be. The Etheric Body will work with the Physical Body to do the work. However, this work may take much time and may or may not be successful, as much depends on how far advanced the problem is before Bio-Etheric Healing began. In any case, repetition of this procedure is needed on a monthly basis for results to be possible.

In the case of tooth problems related to a calcium deficiency, it is wise to examine your diet to minimize or avoid white flour (processed) products and sugar in its many forms. The addition of a multivitamin and mineral formula, as well as calcium and magnesium on a two-to-one ratio of calcium to magnesium is recommended. These should be taken in a chelated and elemental tablet form for better absorption. Also, the addition of vitamin C will be helpful for teeth and particularly the gums. You can ask the Etheric Body, using your Communication Skills, to see how much calcium/magnesium and vitamin C is needed. The Etheric Body can also help heal gum problems when asked to do so.

At the same time, as the Throat Chakra (#5) is involved with the metabolism of calcium, it is wise to ask your Etheric Body if the Throat Chakra or its vortices are cloudy, out of balance, or blocked. Then, ask your Etheric Body to clear, balance, or unblock these as needed. This should help normalize calcium metabolism in the body as a support to healthier teeth.

TRAUMAS (PAST OR PRESENT LIFE)

Traumas are a disordered psychic or behavioral condition in an individual, usually as a result of mental or emotional stress and/or physical injury. Traumas represent a critical challenge to one's ability to function normally without undergoing concentrated psychological and possibly physical rehabilitation therapy. Memory of a Trauma of present, and even past lives, reside in the Mental Body of the Aura. Until and unless the Trauma is dealt with, the accompanying stress (fear, anxiety, et cetera) is still present and affects the body negatively, often insidiously. This stress can work directly to create other health problems, such as ulcers, pain, and phobias. It also works indirectly to play a role in other health problems by interfering with the proper functioning of the immune system and also of the Heart Chakra (#4). These indirectly-affected problems include such auto-immune diseases as colitis, rheumatoid arthritis, and lupus erythematosus. (See separate sections on each of these diseases.)

When these health problems and others, including pain or strange behavior patterns, do not seem to respond to any known treatment, then it is possible that its cause or origin may be due to Trauma(s) residing in the Mental Body of the Aura.

The important first step, and prerequisite to dealing with these diseases, is to get the Trauma (and therefore its harmful effects) out of the Mental Body of the Aura. To do this, ask the Etheric Body separately, for the present life and for past lives, if there is any Trauma involved in the specific illness or disease in question. If a Trauma is involved, for present or past lives or both, you must ask removal for each one separately. Ask the Etheric Body to remove the Trauma involved in the disease out of the Mental Body. However, before making this request, you must first get permission from the Soul to do so. If permission is not granted, do not proceed, as the Trauma may be serving a useful purpose by acting as a safety valve, protecting us from other life-threatening situations in our present lives.

If permission is granted by the Soul and you act to remove the Trauma as discussed above, be forewarned that most likely there will be detoxification symptoms as a result. This detoxification can take many forms, including severe energy depletion, increased heartbeat rate, an upset digestive system, and colds or skin eruptions, as well as temporary worsening of symptoms. There may be no such symptoms, but it is best to be aware of the possibility because these symptoms are a natural part of detoxification.

There may be more than one Trauma involved in a particular disease from present life, but more likely from past lives. Therefore, after removing any indicated Trauma on an initial go-round, it is wise to go back to the first step to ask the Etheric Body again, for both present and past lives separately, if there is any other Trauma involved with the specific disease or illness. If so, you need to repeat the entire procedure described above to remove this additionally involved Trauma. However, be sure to allow a time lapse of a week before asking for removal of additional Traumas. The more deep-rooted the Trauma is, the more difficult its removal from the

Mental Body. You can use your Communication Skills to ask the Etheric Body if a Trauma is finally out, and ask again if it is ready to work on another Trauma.

ULCERS (STOMACH)

Ulcers are an open sore in the lining of the stomach or upper intestine which tend not to heal, causing pain, especially after eating solid food. Stomach ulcers should always be taken seriously because of the danger of hemorrhage and perforation, possibly followed by peritonitis. Ulcers are caused by chemical reactions in the body to extended psychological stress from such conditions as anxiety, tension, overwork, feelings of rejection, anger, or of helplessness, et cetera.

It is wise to seek the help of a medical professional for a full evaluation of the condition, its treatment and suggestions for a special diet, customized to the level of severity of the condition. Also, consider ways to avoid the conditions causing the stress, or if this is not possible, ways which can help you deal with it appropriately. Psychological counseling may be advisable. As serious stress, in its many forms, always affects the Heart Chakra (#4), Bio-Etheric Healing may be of important help. Ask the Etheric Body to balance the Heart Chakra and its vortices. This should normalize its flow of energy and prevent any overactivity. Then, ask the Etheric Body to neutralize the acidity level in the body. Also ask the Etheric Body to clear the Emotional Body and to help calm it. Repeat as often as necessary, possibly on a regular weekly or even daily basis.

Stomach ulcers may also involve the Solar Plexus Chakra. Therefore, it is wise to check if this chakra is blocked, cloudy or unbalanced. If any of these problems exist, ask the Etheric Body to treat accordingly.

VERTIGO

Vertigo is a condition of dizziness and inability to maintain one's equilibrium. It can result from a very wide variety of causes. These range from rapidly moving objects followed by the eyes, looking down from heights, sudden changes in body position, seasickness, intoxication, injuries and infections of the ears and also of the brain, and auditory nerve disorders.

In many cases of vertigo, there is involvement of the Throat Chakra (#5) and its vortices. The involvement is a blockage of energy in this chakra. Ask the Etheric Body if the Throat Chakra is involved in your particular case of vertigo. If it is, ask the Etheric Body to break up the blocked energy in this chakra and its vortices.

YEAST INFECTION (CANDIDA)

Candida is a parasitic fungus that resembles yeast. Once entrenched in the body, it is difficult to overcome. An important element in its control is dietary. You must eliminate all sugars or sweeteners in any form, all yeasted flour products (such as bread, rolls, et cetera), all fermented products (such as beer, wine, liquor, et cetera), all pickled products, and mushrooms in any form, until the infection is gone.

As the fungus is a lower form of life, it is part of the group of life forms that are governed by the Devic Kingdom. (See Chapter VI, "The Devic Kingdom and its Role in Bio-Etheric Healing.") Therefore, it becomes possible to get rid of the infection by dealing with the Deva who oversees the yeast infection or candida. Ask to speak to this Deva. Remember, you may contact the Deva using Inner Speaking, and if you haven't mastered Inner Listening, her answers can come to you via Kinesiology, Head Motions, or Radiesthesia. Once communication is established, be friendly but respectful, as Devas like to have friendly conversations with people who ask work of them. Ask the Deva of Candida to remove the yeast infection from your body. Remember to be cordial and thank her for what she is doing for you. Say "goodbye" and tell her you will contact her again in a few weeks.

After that time, even if you feel better, contact her again by asking to speak to her. Thank her for working with you and ask if the fungus is completely out of your body. If not, ask her again to please work to remove it completely and thank her again. Make contact as many times as you need to in order to get free of the fungus.

Chapter IX

CASE HISTORIES IN BIO-ETHERIC HEALING

This chapter is to chronicle some of the actual real-life experiences of applying Bio-Etheric Healing with adults and children for specific ailments. These case histories have been prepared by the author based on her contemporary notes of the events.

All the case histories have been prepared with the permission of the people involved, and in the case of children, with their parents or guardian. In many cases, letters from the parties involved have been received acknowledging the healing and attesting to its success. These letters have also provided useful information for the case histories. Where permission has been granted, these letters are also included in whole, or edited for the sake of brevity. Also, actual names and initials have been changed to protect the privacy of these individuals.

These case histories and letters have been selected for inclusion to provide added insight into this new concept by illustrating the experiences of people with it, as well as the wide range and unique nature that these experiences exhibit. It is also meant to illustrate that there exist yet unknown and perhaps unknowable possibilities to the experiences and promising opportunities of this breakthrough healing method.

These are the more significant case histories which are completed and available for release at the time of this writing. Other cases, covering more pedestrian situations of pain (headache, body aches, and dental pain), as well as other relatively minor ailments, though no less important to the sufferer, are not included here. Still other case histories of significant healing exist but are not available at this time because a release has not yet been approved or received.

The case histories that follow are presented separately for those involving adults and for infants and children. Also included are two cases of work with Karma that are not health related.

CASE HISTORIES — ADULTS

CASE HISTORY #1

Colitis	November, 1993
Healing Work From A Distance	Boardman, OH

This is a case of a lovely young woman, BHJ, who had a history of colitis for 25 years prior to 1993, when she first asked me to work with her. She called me quite upset, as she had recurring attacks of colitis most of her adult life and lived in fear of these attacks continuing for the rest of her life. The ailment was also a financial drain, as the medications are very expensive.

BHJ gave me permission to use Bio-Etheric Healing to work with her colitis, and the healing work began. I contacted her Etheric Body and asked it to get the disease of colitis, as well as the Miasm of the disease, out of her body.

I remembered that previously Kwan Yin had channeled to me the information that fear is a basic cause of colitis and that fear works to block the Heart Chakra. I asked BHJ's Etheric Body to free the blocked energy of her Heart Chakra. Then I asked that the Traumas of past and present lives relating to the colitis be removed from her Mental Body (after first getting the necessary permission from BHJ's Soul that it was safe to do this.)

I also cleared any current anxiety which BHJ might be experiencing by asking her Etheric Body to clear her Emotional Body. In order to maintain this progress, I taught BHJ how to do this latter work, as well as the basic concept and procedures of Bio-Etheric Healing, especially those related to colitis. This young woman is now able to work with her Etheric Body to maintain her good health. In fact, she can talk to her Etheric Body and get a voice response.

BHJ has been in a state of remission for over three years as of this writing. In her own words, "It is a wonderful feeling to know that I no longer have colitis."

Here is the complete text of her letter:

Dear Mrs. Lanitis:

Some time ago, I had spoken to you about my severe problem with colitis which I have had for about twenty-five years. We spoke about your method of Bio-Etheric Healing as a possibility to help me with this problem. I gave you permission to work with me with Bio-Etheric Healing.

I am most happy that you have decided to write a book about Bio-Etheric Healing to tell others about it. The results of it for me have been wonderful. Shortly after working together on this my colitis began to clear up and I am happy to report that it has been in remission for three years now. I have never had it in remission this long before.

Thank you so much for helping. I cheerfully give you permission to use this letter as a testimonial of my experience.

Yours truly,
BHJ

CASE HISTORY #2

Lyme Disease	August, 1994 High Falls, NY

A neighbor, GR, suspected she had Lyme disease and asked me about it. I tested her using Kinesiology and was saddened to find that she tested positive. This result was further confirmed by symptoms which followed the pattern for this disease. She was feeling sluggish, had arthritic-like pain in her hands, feeling feverish, and also remembered having had the early telltale sign of the red rash associated with Lyme disease.

She gave me permission to work with her using Bio-Etheric Healing. I began working with her Etheric Body immediately, knowing the importance of removing the toxins of Lyme disease from her body.

It should be noted here that several years earlier I myself contracted Lyme disease and had learned of an important aspect to this ailment. Lyme disease is a member of the syphilis family. Like syphilis, it has a bacteria called a spirochete. These spirochetes have a facility to hide in the soft tissue of the body. When antibiotics are used, as is the usual treatment, they cannot reach the spirochetes that are hidden in the soft tissue. As a result, these spirochetes survive and are able to emerge at any time throughout a person's lifetime. They can cause a return of the disease and are a constant threat unless they are all completely removed or annihilated.

In my own experience with Lyme disease, before my development of Bio-Etheric Healing, I had worked with the Deva of the deer tick to get rid of the spirochetes from the soft tissue of my body. It worked, but it was a long process, lasting several months.

In this case, the first time I had worked with someone else who had Lyme disease, I simply asked her Etheric Body to destroy the bacteria of the Lyme disease (the spirochetes), and get them all out of her body.

Next, I asked GR's Etheric Body to clear her Physical Body of all the symptoms which accompanied the Lyme disease, and to restore her to good health.

I then instructed GR to drink a lot of water to help clear her body of toxins as an aid to the expected detoxification process.

I contacted GR's Etheric Body about a week later to see how the healing work was progressing. Her Etheric Body reported that all the spirochetes were now out of GR's Physical Body. I asked if that included the spirochetes in the soft tissue as well, and the response was "Of course." I thanked her and said "Goodbye."

GR is a very spiritual person and she asked me to teach her all about Bio-Etheric Healing and how to do it. I worked with GR for quite a while as she was so eager to use it for self-help and for helping her family. She used it with her brother, sister, and even her dog to rid them of Lyme disease as well.

GR has written an extensive letter describing her experience with and reaction to Bio-Etheric Healing. Excerpts from her letter follow:

> In mid-August of 1994, I woke one morning and noticed a red oval mark, about 2″ wide and 5″ long, above my knee on my left inner thigh…the mark remained for about four more days before it was gone. As the days went on, I was much more easily fatigued than usual. I often woke up…drenched with sweat. During the day I was full of aches and pain twinges, plus I was aware of a

"fever feeling" around my eyes. I suspected Lyme disease, as I had visited my brother in Oak Beach, on Long Island, which is known for a high deer tick count.

Shortly after recognizing that this might be a progression of Lyme disease, I spoke to my sister on Long Island, who seemed to have the same symptoms and was planning to get a blood test for Lyme disease. I had a lapse of medical coverage, and couldn't afford the expense of a blood test. I told my sister I would talk to Trudy about healing us. My sister wanted to go on antibiotics, though they usually give her side effects.

The next day I saw Trudy and told her about my conviction of having Lyme disease. We used Kinesiology to confirm the diagnosis for myself and my sister. Trudy asked my permission to use Bio-Etheric Healing, her method, to heal me, and I immediately consented (since I wanted to ask her exactly that, please)... I then asked Trudy to teach me how to use it to heal my sister.

So Trudy worked with my Etheric Body that night. The next day I felt lighter, more clear headed, not achy or feverish. The day after that I felt energized. It was a very calm feeling of being and becoming stronger.

I was worked on by Trudy on a Wednesday. On Friday I was "un-fatigued" enough to do Bio-Etheric Healing on my sister. When I talked to her on Saturday, she said she felt better, no aches or fever, but was sleeping a lot...she had already started her antibiotics without a blood test, at her doctor's suggestion. At Trudy's suggestion, I used Bio-Etheric Healing on my sister again, this time to ask her Etheric Body to mitigate the side effects she usually has when taking antibiotics. I did this two days in a row. I spoke to her a few days later, and she sounded as if she had never been sick. She was surprised the medicine hadn't made her tired... I am convinced that Trudy has discovered a very viable way of healing, and that she is well on the way to developing a clear process for teaching this method to others.

Sincerely,
GR
High Falls, NY

CASE HISTORY #3

Spinal Disc Regeneration	June, 1993-February, 1995
	McKinney, TX

This is a case concerning my own son, Philip, who lives in the Dallas area.

Philip had been athletic all his life, and played a lot of football in particular. In the late 1980's, he began suffering from back pain and began taking painkillers for relief. He found himself taking so many painkillers that he, himself, was concerned. However, it was the only way he could get through his active schedule as a sales executive.

His MRI tests revealed that three discs of his lower spine were totally missing. He refused to have surgery to fuse his spine and was in acute pain most of the time.

As I developed Bio-Etheric Healing and became more aware of what it was able to accomplish, I was eager to see if it could help him. I was not sure whether it would work for him, and I told him so, but he gave me his permission to try.

I contacted his Etheric Body (over the distance to the Dallas area from the East Coast where I live) and I asked if it could regenerate the missing discs. His Etheric Body was willing to try. Using the Bio-Etheric Healing procedure for reconstructive work, I asked his Etheric Body to use the 7th layer of the Aura, the Ketheric Template, as a guide to what healthy discs would look like. I asked his Etheric Body to work with this guide, or blueprint, and to try to regenerate them where they were missing.

Over the next year, I contacted my son's Etheric Body to repeat the request and to see if any progress was being made. The second time I made the contact, about nine months after my original request, his Etheric Body informed me that the work was progressing and that the discs were halfway finished. It said that he would soon have three regenerated discs in his spine.

Some time later, my son informed me that he had no more back pain and that he was feeling so good that he had begun playing touch football, volleyball, and golf, and was resuming his normal, active life.

Following is the complete text of his letter:

February 20, 1995

Dear Mom:

Hope all is well with you both and that you are enjoying
a warm winter in Florida. Per your request, it is with
great ease that I write this letter concerning your ability
to help with my ailing back.

I first started with problems in 1983. The original
diagnosis by the medical profession was back spasms. I
could not believe how a fluttering muscle could cause
such severe pain. I have used every pain, muscle relaxer
and anti-inflammatory medication known to mankind.
I have spent two weeks in traction and countless hours
in physical therapy. I attended classes at the renowned
North Texas Back Institute. All of these treatments
never relieved the pain for any extended period of time
nor allowed me to continue with my active lifestyle. In
1990 an MRI examination determined that I had three
degenerated discs in my lower back and that only
surgery would give me relief. With a TENS unit in
place I started seeking alternatives to the prescribed
surgery.

Alphabiotic techniques offered some extended relief
but nothing compared to what you have been able to
accomplish for me. I have been enjoying a very active
lifestyle again including football, softball and golf. I
really don't know exactly how it works but I do know
that it does work.

I am forever grateful for your help and encourage you
in your continued work with this miracle cure.

Your loving son,
Phil

CASE HISTORY #4

Simple, But Persistent Headaches   **April, 1995**
                                              Kingston, NY

Several of my friends and I have lunch together on a regular
weekly basis. On one such recent occasion, our regular waitress

blurted out that she was having one of her usual persistent headaches, but that it was particularly painful that day.

Taking her aside, I asked her about her problem. It seems that she has been having these headaches quite regularly, and has been using heavier dosages of aspirin lately to combat them. She was concerned that the headaches continued and she was not comfortable with taking so much aspirin. Also, the aspirin wasn't particularly helpful.

I explained a little about Bio-Etheric Healing. She was eager to try it and granted me permission to work with her.

I asked her Etheric Body to break up the blocked energy that was causing the headache. I returned to my friends and lunch.

About fifteen minutes later, the waitress came over to our table with a big, bright smile to announce that her headache was completely gone. She was very happy and wanted to know how I did that.

We arranged another place and time to meet, during which I taught her the basic concept and procedure for her to help herself in the future.

CASE HISTORY #5

Ulcerative Colitis	February, 1995
Healing Work From A Distance	Battle Ground, WA

GEM is a young mother who has had ulcerative colitis for seventeen years, half of her lifetime. She has tried very many therapies, both traditional and alternative, however, the condition had persisted. It was both psychologically and physically debilitating.

GEM heard of my work and called me to see if Bio-Etheric Healing could help her. She granted me permission to work with her Etheric Body.

The communication with her Etheric Body confirmed that the basic cause of her colitis was an unidentifiable fear. Additional diagnostic work with her Etheric Body indicated that this fear was related to Traumas of both present and past lives that needed to be removed.

Following Bio-Etheric Healing procedures, I first asked permission from the Soul before proceeding. I asked GEM's Etheric Body to remove the Traumas of present and past lives related to that fear from her Mental Body as well as her Emotional Body.

Next, it was necessary to clear the blocked energy from the Heart Chakra which her Etheric Body accomplished upon my request.

Finally, to ensure against recurrence of the problem, I asked her Etheric Body to remove the Miasm for colitis out of her body.

The result of all this work was so exciting and heartwarming to GEM. She began to feel better very quickly, and has completely ended her reliance on drugs for relief. She is particularly pleased at the freedom and confidence she enjoys at being able to be out all day doing the normal routine of a young mother.

I have also taught GEM some of the techniques of Bio-Etheric Healing in order for her to deal with any current anxieties that may arise in her daily life. This involves having the Etheric Body clear her Emotional Body when and as often as needed.

Following is the full text of her letter:

> July 25, 1995
>
> Dear Trudy,
>
> Thank you, thank you! I needed to follow up on my original letter to you written shortly after you first began working with me. At that point, it was too soon for me to know if I was truly healed.
>
> Six months have passed since then. What you have achieved by healing my colitis is incredible. I have been symptom-free for that entire time, with one minor exception that you quickly cured when I called you.
>
> I cannot believe how wonderful it feels to know that I am finally free of this debilitating disease that affected by life in so many ways. I had tried so many other methods: acupuncture, antibiotics, homeopathy, nutrition, supplements, hypnosis. None of these worked for long or gave me the peace of mind that I now have in knowing that you are there for me.
>
> I feel once again like a "normal" person. I am so grateful to you. Thank you.
>
> G.E.M.

CASE HISTORY #6

Vision Problems   October, 1994
                                                      Salem, OH

This case concerns a commercial pilot who, for the last six years, had vision of 20/25, which meant that he had to have a pilot's license reading "with limitations." This required him to wear glasses to bring his vision to 20/20.

B.J. was facing the time to renew his commercial flight instructor's license, which required the Federal Aviation Agency's physical exam, including another vision test.

Ten days before this exam, he asked me if Bio-Etheric Healing might be used to improve his vision and if I would try to help him. I was not sure I could help as the time was so short. It was an interesting challenge.

I started immediately by contacting his Etheric Body and asked it to help. His Etheric Body said it would try to see what it could do. I asked for its help to have B.J.'s vision improved to bring his eyesight up to 20/20.

On the day of his exam, B.J. registered 20/20 on his vision test and he received his commercial pilot instructor's license "without limitation."

Following is the complete text of his letter:

March 15, 1995

Dear Mrs. Lanitis,

As a commercial flight instructor, I have to take an FAA physical examination every year to renew my second class medical certificate.

My last examination, in October of 1994, was a pleasant surprise. For the first time in the last six years I was granted the certificate without limitations.

How does this 46 year old aviator explain the improvement in his vision? Bio-Etheric Healing!

This method made all the difference in the world and allowed me to pass with flying colors.

Thank you for sharing your gift with me.

Sincerely yours,
B.J.

CASE HISTORY #7

Ruptured Spinal Discs	January, 1995
Healing Work From A Distance	N. San Juan, CA
Client En Route Between Two Locations	

In January, 1995, our daughter was visiting us where we were vacationing in Florida. One day she received a phone call from her husband that a trucker friend of theirs, P.D., had severe pain in his lower back. My daughter asked if I would help him if he gave me permission.

We corresponded by answering machine, as he was en route in his truck somewhere between Seattle and Los Angeles. The message from him on our machine asked for my help and gave me permission to try using Bio-Etheric Healing. He was in such pain that his wife was now driving the truck while he lay in the cab behind.

We then received a phone call giving us a description of the problem. He had already spent five days in the hospital, had MRI's taken, and was diagnosed as having two ruptured discs in his spine. One had 75% of the matter, and the other 65% of the matter out of the discs and either floating around the body or in the spinal cord. He had been put on painkillers for the excruciating pain and was having ill effects from the painkillers as well.

With him in transit and with no stationary address, I was not sure I could contact his Etheric Body. I asked my Etheric Body for help to connect up with his Etheric Body, giving his name, his home address, and also the geographic area he was traveling within. My Etheric Body was able to make the link much to my surprise and delight of discovery.

Once contact was made, I asked his Etheric Body to collect the vagabond cells and get them back into the discs. At the same time, I told his Etheric Body to strengthen the walls of the discs to hold the cells in place. I also asked that any missing cells be replaced by new cells. Then I asked the Etheric Body to use the 7th layer of the Aura (the Ketheric Template layer) as a guide to what the new cells should be like. Also I asked his Etheric Body to break up the blocked energy that was causing him pain, and to continue doing that day and night around the clock, as long as it was needed.

The next day we received a message on our machine from his wife that "P.D. is awake this morning and feeling so much better that he couldn't believe it. Please keep on doing what you are doing."

A few days later we received another message, "He is improving rapidly."

Within one week he was back to driving his truck and his wife was home again!

Following are excerpts from a lengthy letter from his wife several weeks later:

> P.D. has been a truck driver for fifteen years... Sunday his back became very painful...he drove one thousand miles with the pain. The more he drove the more crooked his spine became. His right hip was sticking out about eight inches past his shoulder. He could hardly walk. He came home Thursday, January 19, 1995, and had already seen his chiropractor. He went back to the chiropractor, and then to a doctor for muscle relaxers. He never could get any relief. Saturday night, January 21st, the pain became so intense, I took him back to the doctor for a shot of Demerol and cortisone. Well, this helped till 3:00 a.m., and 6:00 a.m. where again pain was beyond belief and complete body is in spasms. I begged the doctor to give him a referral to the hospital...
>
> So Sunday we went back to doctor's office for a shot of Demerol, but they were out of it, so they gave him morphine, which P.D. was allergic to. He didn't get any relief; just itchy hives. Meanwhile, P.D.'s legs got numb.
>
> I came home from work and found five of our neighbors were sliding P.D. onto a piece of plywood. They were trying to put him in the back of the Subaru wagon, to go to the hospital. P.D. was in severe pain for twenty-four miles of curvy road. He screamed in agony. At the hospital, they tried to X-ray him, but his spasms were too intense. I thought he was going to bend the rails off his bed, and his eyes popping out of his head... They finally started an I.V. with Demerol, thank God! He also had Demerol and muscle relaxants by mouth. Five days later he was approved for an MRI scan. The doctor informed us that he had two herniated discs in the lower back. One was 75% into the spinal cord; the other was

65% into the spinal cord. I was thinking this is the end of our trucking business... P.D. had spent each day in the hospital in physical therapy, and he still wasn't able to stand up straight, hip sticking out six inches beyond shoulder...

After six days home, P.D. talked me into driving his truck, with him in the sleeper... We had no money and a payment due on the truck. So we left Friday, picked up a load and headed for Salt Lake, Utah. Monday night we received a phone call in our car phone that Trudy might be able to help P.D. We called back and left a message on Trudy's answering machine, "Please help P.D. He wasn't doing real good; still a lot of pain." We called to say the two lowest discs were herniated; one 75%, the other 65% in the spinal cord. We thought no more about it. We were headed for San Jose, and we were in Salem, Oregon. We had a lot of driving to do. Well, the next morning P.D. woke up and said, "You're not going to believe this, but my back hardly hurts'. I said, 'Oh boy, Trudy must have sent the fairies to help you."

We were so excited, we now felt our trucking business had a chance. On Wednesday, we called Trudy and told her how thankful we both were for her healing powers. Every day after, P.D. became a little better. By the following week I was back at home with the family, and P.D. was on the road again by himself. We cannot thank Trudy enough.

We love you, Trudy.

P.D. and E.D.

CASE HISTORY #8

Poison Ivy   May, 1995
                                              Kingston, NY

A young woman (F.T.) who had heard about me from someone I had previously helped, called to see if I could help her with a bad case of poison ivy. She got it while working in her beautiful garden, and as she cannot identify the poison ivy plant easily, she apparently gets infected often.

I had not worked with poison ivy before, and told her so; but she asked me to please teach her the Bio-Etheric Healing techniques that could help her.

We met and I introduced her to the concept of the Etheric Body and how to communicate with it and enlist its cooperation. I then told her to ask her Etheric Body to dry up all the pustules that had already appeared on the surface of her skin. She then was to ask her Etheric Body to prevent any new pustules from coming out.

Very soon after that meeting, F.T. called to tell me that the poison ivy "just went away."

CASE HISTORY #9

Cancer — Supportive Healing Work	February-July, 1995
Relief From Side Effects Of	St. Petersburg, Fl
Chemotherapy And Radiation	

My first workshop in Bio-Etheric Healing in Florida was originally conceived to focus on the problem of the HIV virus. Of the people that attended this workshop, many were healers themselves, some were simply curious, and some had other specific problems for which they sought answers. A few people asked what Bio-Etheric Healing could do for cancer and I gave them a simple version of the possibilities.

One of the people who asked about cancer was a woman seated in the front row; a quiet, small woman with a turban on her head. Next to her was an intense young man who had come with her. She had had surgery for breast cancer which had progressed to her lymph nodes. She was a spiritual healer herself, as well as a psychic, which I discovered later on. The young man was studying to be a healer at New Age Ministries.

A few days after the workshop, I telephoned the woman and suggested a more complete program, tailored to her specific needs, to help support her recovery and provide relief from the debilitating effects of cancer treatments. She was undergoing chemotherapy and would also have radiation. I outlined specific step-by-step Bio-Etheric Healing procedures for her to follow.

About five or six weeks later, I received a phone call from the young man. He told me that he had followed the procedures I had outlined to work with her. She was so very pleased at how much it helped to reduce the debilitating effects of her cancer treatments that she wanted him to let me know how much she appreciated my help. She wanted me to know before I left Florida for home.

Four months later, on August 1, 1995, I received a letter from the young man. He wrote that he had followed the program for the healing support work that I had outlined for the woman. He had been regularly attending her with Bio-Etheric Healing work during many trips to the hospital and her home to work with her. He reported happily that in July, after all her medical treatments, tests showed her to be free of cancer. He also reported that she told him that the illness and the cancer treatments made her so weak and sick, that at times she didn't think she would have survived without the Bio-Etheric Healing work he had administered. It revived her physical strength and energy level between the medical treatments.

Here are excerpts of the letter from the attending healer:

> My first experience in healing was on a female friend from church. She was diagnosed with cancer of the breast and lymph nodes.... Being virtually untrained, my friend was teaching me how to heal when I worked on her, as she was a psychic and healer. We attended one of Trudy's workshops and were impressed with the concepts of the Bio-Etheric process.
>
> My friend got directions from Trudy on how and where to send energy to treat this illness. I followed these steps in healing when I would work on my friend. I made many trips to the hospital and her home for healing sessions. She was also treated with radiation and chemotherapy. There were times in the hospital she told me she didn't think she would have survived without these healings, her illness and treatment made her so sick....
>
> Toward the end of her ordeal, she confessed to me that a year prior to her diagnosis, she decided she no longer wanted to be on the earth plane. This compli-cated her healing process. She did have a change of thought on that matter, thank God....
>
> Finally good news. After all her treatments and heal-ings, tests performed in July 1995 show her free of any cancer....

...when I am able to fully command your technique, I feel the results will be remarkable, perhaps unbelievable. I eagerly anticipate the time when I can more effectively use your technique.

Very truly yours,
G.R.

CASE HISTORY #10

Spinal Bone Separation (Spinal Bifida)	May-July, 1997 Ashokan, NY

This case involves a young woman, E.S., who attended a series of my classes at a nearby college. She was very spiritual and was able to establish contact with her Etheric Body at the very first session. She was anxious to get started on healing a spinal bone separation problem she had since childhood. After class she asked me to help guide her in addressing this problem specifically. This case is remarkable for several reasons: the ease with which E.S. began working with her Etheric Body, the structural nature of her problem, and the completeness of the healing process (there are "before" and "after" X-rays).

Following my instructions, E.S. directed her Etheric Body to the Ketheric Template, which is in the 7th Layer of the Aura, as a guide to what structural repair was needed. She then asked her Etheric Body to do the necessary healing work, repeating her instructions every so often.

The following is the complete text of her letter which describes this special case in her own joyous words:

Dear Trudy,

I am so thankful for participating in your class. For me it has opened new doors for a way of healing. It's easy and once applying Bio-Etheric Healing, it really feels natural. I believe there is the ability to heal within us all. Sometimes, because of society's changing lifestyle, we begin to doubt ourselves. I am excited that more natural ways of healing are returning and am thankful for people like you who are teaching them.

I have used your methods and have cured myself of things as simple as hiccups to healing a separated bone in my lower spine. I have had back pain most of my life. Fourteen years ago, at the age of 15, an X-ray showed a bone separation in the lower part of my spine. I was told it was this way since birth and there was nothing that could be done to help me.

During the first day of your class, I began applying your methods. A few weeks later you told me you received a message that the healing on my back had begun, and that it would take some time, years perhaps, to heal completely.

Soon after I went for another X-ray. I thought that seeing the separation would help me in visualizing exactly what needed to be healed. I was surprised when I was told there was nothing at all abnormal with my back. The X-ray showed no separation.

I have definitely felt a change for the better. The continued nerve pinching I had over the years seems to be gone. I will continue working on strengthening the area being healed. I am careful to not overdo myself and discourage the healing process.

Thank you again for everything.

Sincerely,
E.S.

WORK WITH HIV-POSITIVE INDIVIDUALS

Background Information

Before going into Case History Number 11, it is important to discuss some relevant issues facing those who work with HIV-positive individuals.

In the State of Florida, there seems to be a feeling among many in the medical community regarding retesting for HIV-positive virus, that since there is no cure for the disease, there is no need for people to be retested. This situation is supported in the actual marketplace. Many of the HIV-positive individuals have used up much of their money and are living on disability, Social Security, and Medicaid, and therefore, disinclined to retest, particularly with the tests so expensive.

Therefore, with this environment discouraging retesting for HIV-positive, it has been difficult to collect retest data for evaluating the effectiveness of our work. Recently, a test known as the Burden Viral Load test has been developed which is accepted medically to test for the HIV virus itself. However, this test is relatively expensive, which is an obstacle to its wider use. Other tests of the blood are conducted (platelets, "T-cells," etc.) which monitor the health of the person but do not reveal the presence or absence of the HIV virus. These tests are normally done at six-month and twelve-month intervals.

In the meantime, we are using one of the alternative diagnostic techniques, Kinesiology, which has found some degree of acceptance in medical circles to report on our progress. Kinesiology testing is very promising, and some clients personally have reported improvement in their condition. For example, one has reported reduced muscle spasms and cramps in the extremities and that his abdominal and digestive distress has virtually disappeared. Two mentioned reduced frequency of night sweats.

As of 1996, Bio-Etheric Healing has been used in only a handful of cases. Two of these individuals went on to take the Burden Viral Load Test once it became available and were both found to be free of the virus. Both individuals had the virus for over ten years.

It is important to mention that another factor in the dissemination of information is the delicacy of the issue itself. This requires that the privacy of the individual be respected when they do not wish to go public. In these cases, if allowed, we will use their data with initials only, disguised to protect their identity.

CASE HISTORY #11

HIV-Positive   **1994-1995**
    Florida

RAD is a man in his early forties who has had the HIV virus for over ten years. He is an independent alternative healing professional. He came to my first workshop and was so attuned to the concept and procedures of Bio-Etheric Healing that he attended all my subsequent workshops. He has sought additional personalized instruction and has incorporated this work in his practice, where appropriate.

In the workshops, he emerged as a gifted individual whose curiosity and probing questions helped to add further insights to the magical experience of communicating directly with one's own Etheric Body. He eagerly went to work applying Bio-Etheric Healing techniques to his individual needs. He worked with both his Etheric Body and the Deva of the HIV Virus to rid himself of the virus.

Within eight days of the first workshop, RAD asked for a progress report from the Deva of the HIV Virus and received the wonderful news that the virus was out of his body. This news was almost too good to be readily accepted, and so we sought confirmation. We applied Kinesiology tests and got the same response. We then, individually and separately, contacted his Etheric Body for confirmation and received an affirmative response in each case. As a final step, I contacted Kwan Yin, my spiritual guide, and was delighted (but no longer surprised) at the affirmative response. On his part, RAD applied to his hospital for a Viral Load Burden Test, but was refused. Despite this, RAD was confident of his recovery.

As is the case with HIV-positive patients, there were many other physical symptoms of the disease which existed, such as body pain, night sweats, and muscle spasms. RAD and I worked closely to enlist the help of his Etheric Body to overcome these difficulties. My role was that of coach and cheerleader, teaching and supporting him in this new breakthrough experience of Bio-Etheric Healing. His role was that of athlete, competing to win back his health against an awesome foe. He was committed to this task, and his story perhaps is best told in his own words, quoted, with his permission, from letters he wrote me over a period of time on his progress.

Note: R.A.D. is one of the individuals who took the Burden Viral Load Test in 1996 and was found to be free of the virus.

Here are excerpts from his letters:

May 10, 1995

My Dear Trudy,

Meeting you this year was pure joy in itself, and then learning about your Bio-Etheric Healing work holds me in *AWE!*

I have experienced many quick healings and some things take a few days or so, although now on a continuous basis I sense that subtle positive changes are happening in my overall being all the time. Specifically I want to share how you've helped me and that I am practicing what you taught us in your workshops. This is very often when other methods of healing or meditation didn't or couldn't work....

...Headache and upper abdominal pain (solar plexus) completely gone in less than one minute (and on the phone no less).

...I woke up realizing I had no muscle cramps-spasms in my arms and legs (this had been going on for over a year almost every day!)

...Chronic back pain — *gone!* Even after a big party and all the preparation and moving of furniture. This had been bothering me for years! (This was from months ago, and I'm still fine.)

...Left earache (for months) — *gone!*

...May 1st, 1995 — woke up with left hip pain totally gone — worked all day in a three story house, and did food shopping, all without pain.

...The past week I was experiencing muscle weakness and pain in both legs, the Saturday and Sunday pain in my left hip so bad I could hardly walk. I somehow brought myself to use Bio-Etheric Healing as I went to sleep. *WOW!* I woke up feeling fine.

...I have been able to eliminate or decrease my prescription medication under the direction of my doctors.

...I have also been able to ease up or eliminate some symptoms of cleansing and detoxification of my body....

...I am so excited and grateful about your work. The possibilities seem endless as I let my imagination soar! I look forward to learning and helping others as you continue to guide me in your Bio-Etheric Healing work.

June 9th, 1995

Since May 17th I've been awakened three times with excruciating pain in my knees and elbows. This was deep joint pain that left me unable to hold myself up on my left leg. I finally was able to focus enough to do Bio-Etheric Healing (remembering that you said it works quick with some pain) and the pain was completely gone in a few minutes. It is a week now, and I am completely free of it. Thank you!

July 22, 1995

My Dear Trudy,

I must tell you... I woke up this morning at 5 a.m. knowing that I AM WELL! And I hope to pass on this renewed feeling as I build my whole being to full function!

> Sincerely,
> R.A.D.

CASE HISTORIES — INFANTS AND CHILDREN

CASE HISTORY #12

Teenager	February, 1993-July, 1995
Color Blindness	Kingston, NY
Learning Disabilities	
Allergies	

In 1993, F.A.'s mother told me that her son was color blind. We talked about the possibility of Bio-Etheric Healing helping him, and she gave me her permission to try it. The possibility was not mentioned to him. He was 13 years old.

I began working with F.A.'s Etheric Body at a distance, as I had never met him personally. I verified with the Etheric Body that the cells governing color vision were damaged, which prevented their proper function of discerning color. I knew that work to repair damaged cells was a longer term process requiring repeated requests to the Etheric Body for the necessary healing work.

About a year and a half after I started to work with F.A., I casually asked his mother whether she or he noticed any change in his vision. She told me that he actually was beginning to see color. He had innocently asked if someone could grow out of color blindness, because he, himself, was beginning to discern colors.

At that point, his mother told him about me. He was delighted, and asked if I could help him with his learning disabilities as well. I then asked to meet him so that I might work with him more closely and perhaps teach him some of the techniques of Bio-Etheric Healing. It was good for him to begin to help himself, especially with the longer term, repetitive procedures required for his more difficult problems.

I found him, upon meeting, to be a very handsome and charming teen-ager. He told me how much his improved color vision had helped him in his art class. He could now tell the difference between dark and light green without having to read the labels on the crayons.

I spent time with him teaching him some of the concept and procedures of Bio-Etheric Healing and the communication skills required to speak with the Etheric Body. Then we worked specifically with the healing procedures for learning disability (as described in Chapter VIII under the listing for "Learning Disability"). I gave him instructions on how to do the healing work, particularly the importance of regular repetition. That was in December of 1994.

He has done so well in his studies since then and he says that his report card is the real proof of it. He has passed all his subjects. The summer of 1995 was the first time he was not required to go for remedial work, and thus was able to get a summer job. This achievement, in addition to the knowledge that someone was helping him overcome his problems, helped his confidence grow.

In the spring of 1995, he asked if I could help him with his allergies to pollen. I worked out a program for him and spent some time going over it with him. He was to follow it himself on a self-help basis.

He now reports (July 1995) that as long as he was doing what I had outlined for him, it had worked fine, providing complete relief. For the whole month of June, he was free of symptoms. However, he admits that when he got lazy and stopped the procedures, some of the symptoms began anew. He discovered for himself what I had told him, that repetition of the procedure was required. He has gotten back on track with a three-times-a-week schedule and is enjoying good health.

What a difference Bio-Etheric Healing has made in his young life!

Following is the full text of his mother's letter:

February 8, 1995

Dear Trudy,

My son has been working with you on his color differentiation for one and a half years. Recently he is noticing an improvement, especially in his art class. We both feel that thanks to your great efforts we are seeing an improvement. Please keep up this great spirit and enthusiasm.

Sincerely,
B.A.

CASE HISTORY #13

Ear Infection   November, 1994
                                                        Kingston, NY

A young woman was referred to me who had a one-year-old child, a little girl, suffering from an acute ear infection. The mother was beside herself, as the child screamed in pain night and day. She had been to see the doctor, who put the child on antibiotics, but it didn't seem to help. I offered to try to help the little girl, with her mother's permission. The mother was ready to try anything at that point. Although she had made an appointment to see a specialist, the date was two weeks away.

I worked with the baby over distance, and asked her Etheric Body to kill the bacteria or virus that was causing the infection, and to break up any blocked energy that was causing the pain. I telephoned the mother afterward to inform her I had worked with the child.

A week later I contacted the mother and asked how the baby was, and what had happened. The mother told me that the day after I worked with her daughter, she drank lots and lots of water. (This is an example of detoxification at work.) On the second day she was fine. When the mother subsequently took the child to see the specialist, she was told he could find no signs of anything that could have caused the child's pain and discomfort.

Following is the full text of the mother's letter:

Dear Trudy,   3/31/95

I would like to express our many thanks for you helping our daughter. When she was an infant, she was suffering from continuous bouts with ear infections. I mentioned this to you and you asked if you could try to reach this problem. I was ready and willing to get relief for her.

After your working with her I brought her to a specialist for an opinion and he said her ears looked fine and very healthy.

I again would like to take this time to thank you for your efforts.

Sincerely,
F.T.

CASE HISTORY #14

Work With Newborn To Age Three	1992-1995
Ingestion Of Amniotic Fluid	Stamford, CT
Colic	
Growth Problems	

I first contacted Baby Gerry's Etheric Body, at the request of his grandmother, a few days after he was born. He had gone through a difficult delivery. The medical diagnosis indicated that he had ingested some amniotic fluid. He was in the hospital with tubes inserted in his body. The medical team attending him felt that if he survived he might have serious complications. His grandmother, concerned about his chance of survival, requested that I ask his Etheric Body three questions about his health.

1. "How do you feel?"
2. "Do you want to live?"
3. "If you decide to stay, will you be healthy?"

I did make contact with Baby Gerry's Etheric Body and found its voice very weak. The answers came back very haltingly.

1. "Not good."
2. "I don't know."
3. "I don't know."

At that point, I asked his Etheric Body to help get the amniotic fluid out of his body and to help repair any damage that it may have caused.

About five days later, I contacted Baby Gerry's Etheric Body a second time. He remembered me and said, "Hello Lady." I asked him the same three questions. The response was stronger this time.

1. "I feel better; they treat me real good here."
2. "I may want to live."
3. "I don't know."

When I reported this latest contact to his grandmother, she informed me that the tubes had been removed from his body. The nurses were with him and attentive to his every need.

About five days after the second contact, I contacted Baby Gerry's Etheric Body for the third time. I asked him the same three questions again. Again, he recognized me, and said, "Hello Lady." His voice sounded stronger than before.

1. "I feel better; my mommy and daddy love me, and I love them."
2. "I think I'll live."
3. "I'm not sure if I'll be healthy."

Baby Gerry's grandmother called again when he was three and a half months old to tell me that he had colic. She asked me to contact his Etheric Body to see if I could help. It was wonderful to hear the response from his Etheric Body, even stronger now, and to hear it say, "Hello Nice Lady."

I told Baby Gerry's Etheric Body to break up the blocked energy causing his pain, and to heal and help mature his digestive system. It said it would try and so I said goodbye without too much additional conversation. The colic eased up considerably after that.

When Baby Gerry was three years old, I was again asked by his grandmother to contact his Etheric Body. This time her concern was that he was below average growth and she wanted to see if anything could be done about it.

I did contact Baby Gerry's Etheric Body and it did recognize me immediately again even after so much time had elapsed. (No one else had ever talked to him.) I told him my name was Trudy and asked how he felt. He replied, "I feel pretty good most of the time."

As the Throat Chakra is involved in growth, I asked Baby Gerry's Etheric Body to check his Throat Chakra to see if it was damaged. The response was that one of its vortices was damaged. I then asked his Etheric Body to repair that vortex and to use the Ketheric Template (the 7th layer of the Aura) as a blueprint of what a healthy vortex would look like. The response was that he would try.

I decided to ask little Gerry a question, "Now that you are three years old, how do you feel about yourself?" He answered, "I'm very happy. My mommy and daddy love me, and I love them. Can I call you Lady Trudy, if I want to talk to you? No one else ever tried to talk to me. I like talking to you. Will you call me again?"

I decided to have his Etheric Body check out his chakras and discovered that in addition to the Throat Chakra damage, he had an underactive Sacral Chakra and his Solar Plexus and Third Eye Chakra were blocked and cloudy. I asked his Etheric Body to break up the blocked energy and clear both of the latter two chakras, doing them one at a time. I also asked that it work to balance the Sacral Chakra.

Five days later, I contacted little Gerry's Etheric Body again to see how the healing work was progressing. The response was that the blocked energy of the Third Eye Chakra and the cloudiness were almost gone. Work on the Sacral and Solar Plexus Chakras had not yet begun, but that the repair of the Throat Chakra vortex was well underway.

Little Gerry's Etheric Body also volunteered that the Physical Body was feeling better now that the blockage and cloudiness was being removed.

I decided to ask his Etheric Body some questions:

Question: "When I first contacted you as a newborn, and asked you to heal your Physical Body from the problems incurred during the birth process, were you able to help in the healing?"

Answer: "I don't know if my Physical Body would have been able to survive if you hadn't told me what to do. It is true that the nurses and doctors did everything they could think of to get the amniotic fluid out of my Physical Body, but it was your suggestions to get *me* to start working on the Physical Body that made it possible for the Physical Body to survive. When you first contacted me (the Etheric Body), I was so weak and tired, that I didn't really think I would be able to stay with the Physical Body much longer."

Question: "Do you remember that on a second occasion I talked to you about healing Baby Gerry's colic?"

Answer: "Yes, I do." (At this point, he repeated the same words I used to tell him what to do to help in the healing. He also said that he healed the digestive system, but that took a longer time.)

Two weeks later, I contacted little Gerry's Etheric Body again to see if he had been able to heal the damaged Throat Chakra. His Etheric Body was delighted to hear from me again. "Hello Lady Trudy, Trudy Lady," was the joyous response. "I was able to fix the Throat Chakra, and I think little Gerry will grow much better now that it is fixed."

He then thanked me for alerting him to the problem, and expressed satisfaction in being able to help.

CASE HISTORY #15

Newborn	**October, 1994**
Birth Problems	**Lake Tahoe, CA**
Colic	
Common Cold	

When my grandson was born 3,000 miles from where we live, my husband and I quickly made reservations, packed, and were out at Lake Tahoe in three days. We found a happy, but exhausted, new mother, and her newborn son. The baby boy was adorable. He had a nice head of black hair that stood straight up on his head. We helped in whatever way we could to make things simpler for them.

The baby seemed in obvious discomfort and had been for about a week. I asked my guide, Ignatious, what the problem could be, and he told me that I needed to clear the baby's Astral Body, as well as his Mental and Emotional Bodies. Ignatious said that matter from the mother's Astral Body sometimes attaches to the baby's Astral, Mental, and Emotional Bodies during the birth process. This may make the baby irritable for the first three years of its life. Ignatious also suggested that very often, the chakras get damaged, and sometimes blocked during the birth process.

Therefore, after getting his mother's permission, I asked the baby's Etheric Body to clear the Astral, Mental, and Emotional Bodies of his Aura. He seemed much happier after that. It took several days to do this.

When the baby was about two weeks old, he started to cry and squirm in obvious pain. I checked his Etheric Body to see what could be the matter. He responded positive to colic. I again spoke to his Etheric Body, and asked it to break up any blocked energy (of the chakras) that was causing him pain in his abdomen. After a while his crying and fussing subsided and he seemed much better.

I seemed to have a very good connection via thought-processes with my grandson's Etheric Body. He'd say, "Hello Grammy, Grammy, Grammy," and was really happy to talk to me! He said that from the very first time I contacted his Etheric Body when he was less than a week old.

One day I felt a "PING" on my forehead, and it was my grandson saying, "Hello Grammy, Grammy, Grammy." This was the first time he contacted *me!* It was also the first time that someone else's Etheric Body ever contacted *me!* This tiny, two-week-old baby had an Etheric Body that wanted to talk to *me,* and was able to do so. He said, "Grammy, will you tell my mother what you did to make me feel better so she can make me feel better too?"

I wrote everything out on a piece of paper for my daughter, explaining both the concept and procedures. However, shortly after we returned home to Kingston, New York, I felt his familiar "PING" on my forehead, and there he was — "Hello Grammy, Grammy, Grammy." He told me that he wasn't feeling so good and said, "Grammy, will you teach me to do what *you* do that makes me feel better?" I told his Etheric Body to clear and unblock the chakra points that were giving him pain. He said, "Thank you Grammy, Grammy, Grammy." I always thanked him for contacting me, and told him how very much I loved him. He was three and a half weeks old at that time.

Sometimes he just wants to talk to me, and we have some wonderful conversations. He wants to tell me all about himself, memories of past lives and past experiences.

He knew I was writing a book, and talked about it to me. Unfortunately, I've been so busy with my Bio-Etheric Healing work, that I had less and less contact with him. Also, I thought, perhaps he is getting older and doesn't need me so much. However, I was wrong! He just wanted more meaningful conversations; and now I have a message from him that he wants to include in my book. It is a "message for parents and grandparents."

Here is his message which came on May 26, 1995:

Hi Grammy. I've been looking forward to finding a time to talk to you when you are not in a hurry, or driving your car, or busy with other things. There are so many things I want to talk to you about. I feel very lucky to have a grammy who can hear me and talk back to me. I love you, Grammy. I feel very privileged to have you as my Grammy.

I'm really looking forward to this lifetime. I hope that as a result of your book, Grammy, other mothers and grandmothers will try to reach the Etheric entity that is part of the whole person, the seen and the unseen part.

I would like to tell you more about myself to put into your book. I think other people will want to know about us Etheric Bodies and even you, Grammy. I've talked to you a little bit about it, while you were driving your car. But I want you to write it all down, so you don't forget, and tell others about this. I don't think a seven-and-a-half-month old baby's Etheric Body has ever communicated with the outside world. So it may be of great interest to everyone out there.

We all have lived many lifetimes. We come from the Astral plane, and there's a whole bunch of us who are ready and willing to incarnate at the same time. If we want to, we can choose our parents, from their projected life, this *privilege* is only granted to the very evolved souls. The others have to take whatever body is made available to them and they don't have a choice. It is only after you have reached a certain level of experience and knowledge that you get a chance to choose. So I was granted this opportunity, and chose your family to join. I did know quite a bit about the family, Grammy, and that you were a part of it. I also knew that my mother would be a very loving person, caring for all life forms, and that my father would be a very kind and caring person. So I chose this family.

In early July, 1995, my daughter informed me that my grandson had a cold. I contacted my grandson's Etheric Body and asked it to kill the viruses and bacteria that came into his body. The Etheric

Body answered, "Now I know what they are, and I can do that." A few days later he was fine.

WORKING WITH KARMA — NOT HEALTH RELATED

CASE HISTORIES #16-#17

Background Information

Briefly defined, Karma is a force based upon one's deeds and thoughts acted out in one's lifetime or past lifetimes that determine the consequences of one's current and even future lives. Therefore, one is responsible for his or her Karma and can suffer poor health or bad luck, or conversely, good health or good luck, as a result of how one led his life or lives. In a sense, Karma is an accumulated effect of one's deeds, thoughts, and actions which has affected the past, is affecting the present, and can affect the future of one's life in many ways.

Karma, like the popular concept of "fate," is generally believed to be unchangeable or inescapable. In Hinduism and Buddhism, from which the concept of Karma originated, some means of mitigating or overcoming its effects were possible, primarily through rules of leading a pure life, meditation and chanting.

Bio-Etheric Healing recognizes the potential influence of Karma on a person's current health problems. It discusses ways of working with the Etheric Body to determine if Karma is playing a role, and if so, how to reduce or overcome any negative effects on one's health.

Some of the case histories reported in this chapter, and other illustrations mentioned throughout the book, report on Karmic influence on specific health problems of an individual and how they can be, and have been, overcome. However, the case histories that follow are examples of Karma at work generating frustration, difficulties, and misfortune; in other words, general bad luck unrelated to health. These case histories illustrate how the concept and procedures of Bio-Etheric Healing have worked to overcome the effects of "bad" Karma to provide more gratifying experiences and good fortune.

CASE HISTORY #16

Overcoming Hard Luck	June, 1995-September 1995
Getting The Job Of Your Dreams	Binnewater, NY

S.W. is a very talented and dedicated artist. He lives for his art, but needs to have an outside job to help pay for his rent and food. After twelve years at his job, management and their policies began to change, which made his work life difficult. When the situation became no longer tolerable, S.W. began to seek other employment. After many disappointments in this search, with conditions at work making him more desperate, he and a longtime friend decided to start their own business by pooling their resources, as neither could do it alone.

After working out the details and setting a date, S.W. quit his job and looked eagerly forward to the new joint venture. That same day when he visited his friend to begin work, he found out that his friend (age 39) had suddenly died just a few hours earlier. S.W. was devastated. He had quit his job and he did not have enough resources to carry out the new planned venture alone. He had to conserve his resources for the expected long haul of finding new employment — after experiencing a long, unsuccessful and depressing period of searching.

We met one day, and he recounted his miserable luck and his many unsuccessful job interviews since quitting his job. I suggested that Karma might be at play causing his discouraging situation. After getting his permission, I asked his Etheric Body if Karma was involved, and received a positive response.

I then asked his Etheric Body to break up the Karma causing his bad experiences related to his job and business venture. I asked that this particular Karma be removed from the outer layers of the Aura.

After a wait of two weeks, I contacted S.W.'s Etheric Body again to find out the progress. His Etheric Body responded with excitement and joy and told me that S.W. was going to be offered a wonderful job — the kind he would really like.

I immediately tried to reach S.W. to pass on the good news, but could only get his phone machine. As I wanted to tell him personally, I did not leave a message. It was the following week before I reached him by phone, and as I started to tell him about the wonderful job coming his way, he interrupted to tell me that the job was already his. He had started the previous Wednesday. He was overjoyed. It was the job of his dreams; the job he had always wanted. "How did you do that?" he asked. I told him I would tell him all about Bio-Etheric Healing when we had a little more time together.

Note: In 1996 S.W. was promoted to the headquarters office to serve as a group head, enjoying his work even more. In 1998, he became a freelance consultant serving his old company among other clients and at a higher rate scale.

CASE HISTORY #17

Overcoming A Long String Of Major Business Failures, Not Of One's Own Doing	1983-1995 Dallas, TX

A father of three in his forties, who is a bright, energetic sales executive, had been suffering through twelve years of misfortunes in business. He had started a company which was funded by the capital of two friends who were to be silent partners.

The company grew, and after several years, his reward of a third share partnership for his "sweat equity" was to be conferred. At this point, there erupted a major dispute between the two silent partners and the enterprise was dissolved, leaving the young man empty-handed after so many years of dedication and hard work.

Shortly after that, a second, similar opportunity presented itself to start a business funded by the excess capital and products of a foreign group of entrepreneurs eager to get a foothold in the U.S. market. This time, the proper protection in the form of legal documents were executed to guarantee that he would receive an ownership share of the business at a given point.

A year or so after the business start-up, an assistant for the young man was hired to help with the day-to-day details. Then one day, six months later, our young man arrived at his office to find that the foreign ownership group had "bought" the loyalty of the new assistant, placing him in charge of the company on a salaried basis, and breaking their contractual agreement for an equity share with our young man.

Although he had limited means, our subject brought the case to court and won, accepting a cash settlement in order to get on with his life, rather than face a protracted legal battle.

After struggling to find new employment, our subject joined a small firm which needed an experienced hand to land a contract with a major corporation. His contribution won the contract and a chance to build a business. This time he was starting with an ownership position, using his cash settlement. The business grew steadily.

Soon the business reached a critical mass with investments made in new equipment, facilities, and manpower. New capitalization was needed for further expansion. This rapid success and the amounts of capital needed and the risks involved made the original partner extremely nervous and he asked to be bought out. This came at the worst possible time.

Our subject stretched his resources to buy out his partner just at the time when unforeseen economic troubles began brewing. The economy of Texas took a nose dive. Credit approvals by the corporate client were severely tightened. This resulted in a large proportion of sales already consummated being disapproved. This latter situation was a telling blow and pushed our subject into business and personal bankruptcy.

The bad luck at business continued. After many months of unemployment, he took a lower level sales job which offered some hope of advancement. Within the year, his talents were recognized and rewarded with a promotion to manager of a division of the company. However, his bad Karma exhibited itself again because in less than a year, he was caught in a reorganization and was suddenly let go.

He has now started again, hired by a very successful friend, who asked him to help grow his company in a new direction. The time horizon for succeeding in this objective was expected to be several years. As a result of his demoralizing past experiences, he was feeling that "bad luck" would follow again. That is when he spoke to me about his feelings.

I suggested that I might see if Karma was involved in his business life. He had never heard of Karma, but gave me permission to work with his Etheric Body.

I contacted his Etheric Body, and it confirmed that Karma was blocking his success and causing his unusual difficulty in the business world. I then asked his Etheric Body to break up the bad Karma related to his business life and to rid it from the two outer layers of the Aura.

After two weeks, I asked our subject if he noticed any difference, but he did not. I contacted his Etheric Body again to ask it what was happening. It told me that his bad Karma related to business was so thick that it would take more time to get it dissolved and removed.

About two weeks after that, I received a phone call from our subject. He was so excited at what was happening. He had received a "whole bunch" of orders with some from major national corporations. He asked, "Could it be the Karma?" I told him it probably was and that we should wait to see further evidence of a changed fortune.

A short time later, I got another call that so many of the leads he developed were coming through with purchase orders. His friend and employer was extremely pleased. They were developing strong personal and business ties. Also, his new confidence was establishing strong client relationships. He began calling me regularly with more good news.

After about a year, he received a lucrative offer from a major manufacturer as their key agent representing them to a large multi-industry market for their products. He took this offer and negotiated a contract which allows him to continue developing his own sales organization.

As of 1998, our subject has had considerable success setting up ongoing deals with several national corporations for his new employers. Also, his own personal sales organization has grown very successfully, beyond even his own expectations, assuring him of the financial independence that had previously eluded him. He feels so overjoyed that the spell has been broken finally.

USEFUL ANALYTIC AND
RECORDING WORKSHEETS

On the following pages are three worksheets for suggested use in healing work with yourself or with others. They are meant both as a general guide to gather necessary analytic information, and also as a help in recording that information. In this way, appropriate records are available to guide the healing and its progress over time.

These worksheets are:

1. some basic analytical questions to ask of the person and his/her Etheric Body
2. a worksheet to record instructions given to the Etheric Body
3. an analysis chart of the main Chakras and their vortices (to be conducted periodically, over time, to help keep track of progress)

EVALUATION QUESTIONS

Ask of Person:

- What are all the physical problems you are experiencing with this particular ailment or complaint?
- What, if any, are the emotional problems you are aware of related to this particular ailment or complaint? (When working with another person, try to develop as much information as possible with prompts such as, "What else?")

Ask of the Etheric Body:

- Is this illness related to blocked energy?
- Is this illness related to a chakra problem?
- Is this illness related to a glandular problem?
- Is this illness related to anxiety/fears or psychological aspects?
- Is Karma involved in this particular ailment or complaint? How is it involved? Discover any important nuances.
- Are Traumas of past or present lives implicated? Explore to identify the Trauma and how it is related to this particular ailment or complaint. Ask if there are other Traumas implicated in this same problem?
- Is there a Miasm related to this problem that needs to be removed?
- Are parasites of any kind (in the Physical Body) a causative factor?
- Is there a viral or bacterial infection currently in the Physical Body? Is there a virus present from past illnesses?
- Are there cancer cells in the body? (Ask questions to establish the location.)
- Is there a reason to hold onto this illness?
- Nutritional issues to explore:
  - Acid/alkaline ratio of body
  - Need for calcium magnesium
  - Need for vitamins
  - Existence of free radicals in the body

RECORD OF INSTRUCTIONS GIVEN

Date   Instructions

ANALYSIS CHART OF THE MAIN CHAKRAS
AND THEIR VORTICES

	Blocked	Damaged	Cloudy	Out of Balance
date				
chakra 7				
6				
5				
4				
3				
2				
1				
alta major				
spleen				

✓ = needs work   o = okay   x = improving

NOTES:

EPILOGUE

ABOUT KWAN YIN

Kwan Yin is a deity that has been a Guardian of the Planet Earth for thousands of years. She has played various roles during her time spent on this planet. Among them, she has been the receiver and caretaker of the Violet Flame, which is the source of high energy for the Planet Earth. She has also been the Chohan for the Seventh Ray for 16,000 years, and passed that on to St. Germaine in 1954. She is also a member of the Karmic Board, and is a representative for the Sixth Ray to that Board.

Her work on the Planet Earth is to bring health and mercy to the people of the world.

Best known in the Orient, where she has been revered for thousands of years, she is now more universally known for her work in healing, and bringing healing modalities long known in the Far East to Western civilizations. Some of these modalities have been practiced in the Orient for thousands of years.

She and the Blessed Virgin Mary share a common goal, that is, to bring better health to our planetary residents. She has been compared to other goddesses and healers in the past, but she is unique in the scope of her work and her connections to the Karmic Board. She stands alone in the world with the number of years of service she has given to our planet. It is said that she is the Mother of the Planet, and that without her energy, there would be no life possible on the Earth.

We salute her for the love that she has bestowed upon us, and we love her dearly.

ABOUT LORD KUTHUMI

Lord Kuthumi is known as a master teacher. As such, he is in charge of peace and healing for our Earth, a goal which he shares with Kwan Yin. He was in charge of the Fifth Ray for 14,000 years. His mission now is to seek out those that have a commitment to help humanity, on the Earth plane, and encourage them to bring this work to a broader audience. He wishes to improve the quality of life of the people of the Earth.

Lord Kuthumi is spirit. He has never had a lifetime on this Earth. He works with, and is under the direction of Sanat Kumara, who is Lord of the World. He also works under the command of "The One Above All."

Lord Kuthumi is particularly interested in bringing attention to the great potential for the world that Bio-Etheric Healing holds.

Lord Kuthumi lives among the mists and mountains of Tibet, yet he is always accessible when and where needed. On September 15, 1996, Lord Kuthumi bestowed the title of "Master Healer" to Trudy Lanitis, for her work in developing Bio-Etheric Healing.

ABOUT IGNATIOUS (1924-1941)

Ignatious is spirit, but has spent many lifetimes on Planet Earth. During his last incarnation, he was a childhood friend of Trudy Lanitis, and also had occasion to meet her grandfather, who is now known as the Guardian Angel Hammond. When Ignatious heard that Kwan Yin was helping Trudy to write her book on Bio-Etheric Healing, he volunteered to help Kwan Yin. He subsequently channeled Trudy Lanitis healing directions for some of the illnesses that she was concerned about. He is very happy to have been of service in bringing this knowledge to the Earth plane, and working with Kwan Yin.

ABOUT EDGAR CAYCE (1877-1945)

Although Edgar Cayce is now in spirit, he has had many lifetimes on this earth. In his last incarnation, he was a famous mystic and healer. While in a hypnotic trance, self-induced, he was able to diagnose a person's illnesses and offer solutions, whether a person was far away or close by. He loved his Bible and God, and his life was a struggle to keep his healing work pure and elude those who were trying to take advantage of his innocence and talent for their own profit.

Edgar Cayce discovered Trudy Lanitis' healing work very early on before she had fully developed Bio-Etheric Healing. He felt that he wanted to help her, and he also felt a close relationship to her. They have had many past lifetimes where their lives were interconnected. He started channeling to her in 1991, and was the first to suggest that she would write a book on healing. The book was started, at the urging of Kwan Yin, in February of 1994. Edgar Cayce wanted to be a part of it. He subsequently channeled some of the material included in this book.

BIBLIOGRAPHY

Andrews, Lynn V. *The Medicine Woman*. New York: Harper & Row, 1982.

Angelo, Jack. *Your Healing Power — A Comprehensive Guide to Channeling Your Healing Energies*. London, England: Judy Piatkus Ltd., 1995.

Bailey, Alice A. *A Treatise on White Magic*. New York: Lucis Publishing Co., 1979.

Bailey Alice A. *Esoteric Healing*. New York: Lucis Publishing Co., 1953.

Bailey, Alice A. *Esoteric Psychology*. New York: Lucis Publishing Co., 1970.

Blavatsky, Helena P., Translator. *The Voice of the Silence*. Wheaton, IL: The Theosophical Publishing House, 1992.

Blofeld, John. *Bodhisattva of Compassion — The Mystical Tradition of Kwan Yin*. Boston: Shambhala Publications, 1988.

Brennan, Barbara Ann. *Hands of Light*. New York: Bantam Books, 1987.

Burmeister, Helen S. *The Seven Rays Made Visible*. Marina Del Rey, CA: DeVorss & Company, 1986.

Burmeister, Mary. *Jin Shin Jyutsu — Getting to Know (Help) Myself*. Scottsdale, AZ: Jin Shin Jyutsu, Inc., 1992.

Cayce, Edgar. *Auras*. Virginia Beach, VA: ARE Press, 1945.

Cayce, Edgar. Channeled information to Trudy Lanitis. 1994-1995.

Charlton, Hilda. *Pioneers of the Soul*. Woodstock, NY: Golden Quest, 1992.

Charlton, Hilda. *Saints Alive*. Woodstock, NY: Golden Quest, 1989.

Diamond, John, M.D. *Your Body Doesn't Lie*. New York: Warner Books/Harper & Row, 1978.

DeRohan, Ceanne. (Channeled) *Healing and Evolving the Emotional Body*. Albuquerque, NM: One World Publications, 1987.

The Findhorn Community. *Faces of Findhorn — Images of a Planetary Family*. New York: Harper & Row, 1980.

Garfield, Laeh Maggie and Grant, Jack. *Companions in Spirit*. Berkeley, CA: Celestial Arts, 1984.

Guiley, Rosemary E. *Harper's Encyclopedia of Mystical and Paranormal Experience*. San Francisco, CA: Harper-Collins, 1995.

Halifax, John, Ph.D. *Shamanic Voices*. New York: E.D. Dutton, 1979.

Harner, Michael, Ph.D. *A Guide to Power and Healing, The Way of the Shaman*. New York: Bantam Books, 1986.

Hartman, Jane E., N.D., Ph.D. *Shamanism for the New Age — A Guide to Radionics and Radiesthesia*. Placitas, NM: Aquarian Systems, Inc., 1987.

Hawken, Paul. *The Magic of Findhorn*. New York: Harper & Row, 1975.

Hay, Louise L. *You Can Heal Your Life*. Santa Monica, CA: Hay House, 1987.

Horan, Paula, Ph.D. *Empowerment Through Reiki*. Wilmont, WI: Lotus Light Publications, 1992.

Ignatious. Healing Spirit, Channeled Information on Healing to Trudy Lanitis (1994-1995).

Joy, W. Brough, M.D., *Joy's Way — A Map for the Transformational Journey*. Los Angeles: J.P. Tarcher, Inc., 1979.

Kilner, Walter J., M.D. *The Human Aura*. New York: Samuel Weiser, Inc., 1973.

Krieger, Doris. *The Therapeutic Touch.* Englewood Cliffs, NJ: Prentice Hall, 1979.

Kwan Yin, Goddess of Healing and Compassion for our Planet. Channeled Information on Healing to Trudy Lanitis, 1994-1995.

Lacerda de Azevedo, José, M.D. *Spirit & Matter: New Horizons for Medicine.* Tempe, AZ: New Falcon Publications, 1997.

Lansdowne, Z.F., Ph.D. *Ray Methods of Healing.* York Beach, ME: Samuel Weiser, Inc., 1993.

Levine, Stephen. *A Gradual Awakening.* Garden City, NY: Anchor Books, Doubleday, 1979.

Levition, Richard. *The Imagination of Pentecost.* Hudson, NY: Anthroposophic Press, 1994.

Long, Max Freedom. *The Secret Science at Work — The Huna Method as a Way of Life.* Marina Del Ray, CA: DeVorss & Company, 1991.

Lord Kuthumi, Channeled Information on Healing to Trudy Lanitis, 1994-1995.

Macrae, Janet, Ph.D., R.N. *Therapeutic Touch — A Practical Guide.* New York: Alfred A. Knopf, 1988.

Monahan, Evelyn M. *The Miracle of Metaphysical Healing.* West Nyack, NY: Parker Publishing Co., 1975.

Ostrander, S. and Schroeder, L. *Psychic Discoveries Behind the Iron Curtain.* Englewood Cliffs, NJ: Prentice Hall, 1970.

Padmakara Translation Group. *Shantiveda — The Way of the Bodhisattva.* Boston, MA: Shambala Publications, Inc., 1997.

Prophet, Mark L. and Prophet, Elizabeth C. *Lords of the Seven Rays — Mirror of Consciousness.* Livingston, MT: Summit University Press, 1986.

Roman, Sanaya and Parker, Duane. *Opening Up To Channel.* Tiburon, CA: H.J. Kramer, Inc., 1984.

Russell, Edward W. *Report on Radionics.* England: C.W. Daniel Company, Ltd., 1991.

Stone, Hal, Ph.D. and Winkleman, Sidra, Ph.D. *Embracing Ourselves — Voice Dialogue Manual.* Marina Del Rey, CA: DeVorss & Company, 1985.

Sugrue, Thomas. *The Story of Edgar Cayce, There is a River.* Virginia Beach, VA: ARE Press, 1994.

Tansley, David V., D.C. *Radionics and the Subtle Anatomy of Man.* Devon, England: Health Science Press, 1988.

Tansley, David V., D.C. *Chakras, Rays and Radionics.* Essex, England: C.W. Daniel Company, Ltd., 1984-1992.

Tansley, David V., D.C. *The Raiment of Light — A Study of the Human Aura.* London: Arkana, 1987.

Trungpa, Chogyam. *Shambhala, the Sacred Path of the Warrior.* New York: Bantam Books, 1986.

Wright, Machaelle Small. *Behaving As If The God In All Life Mattered.* Jeffersonton, VA: Perelandra, 1987.

Young, Alan. *Spiritual Healing — Miracle or Mirage?* Marina Del Ray, CA: DeVorss & Company, 1981.

BIBLIOGRAPHY — NUTRITION

Abrahamson, E.M., M.D. and Pezet, A.W. *Body, Mind and Sugar.* New York: Avon Books, 1977.

Adams, Ruth and Murray, Frank. *The Vitamin B-6 Book.* New York: Larchmont Books, 1980.

Cheraskin, E., M.D., D.M.D. and Ringsdorf, W.M., JR., D.M.D. and CLARK, J.W., D.D.S. *Diet and Disease.* New Canaan, CT: Keats Publishing Co., 1977.

Davis, Adele, A.B., M.S. *Let's Eat Right to Keep Fit.* New York: Harcourt, Brace and World, Inc., 1954.

Davis, Adele, A.B., M.S. *Let's Get Well.* New York: Harcourt, Brace and World, Inc., 1965.

Donsbach, Kurt W., Ph.D., D.Sc. *Nutrition In Action.* Huntington Beach, CA: International Institute of Natural Health Sciences, 1979.

Editors of Prevention Magazine. *The Complete Book of Vitamins and Minerals for Health.* Emmaus, PA: Rodale Press, 1988.

Fredericks, Carlton, Ph.D. *New and Complete Nutrition Handbook. Your Key To Good Health.* Huntington Beach, CA: International Institute of Natural Health Sciences, Inc., 1977.

Hoffer, Abram, M.D., Ph.D. and Walker, Morton, D.P.M. *Nutrients To Age Without Senility.* New Canaan, CT: Keats Publishing, Inc., 1980.

Kugler, Hans J., M.D. *Dr. Kugler's Seven Keys to a Longer Life.* Briarcliff Manor, NY: Scarborough House, 1978.

Null, Gary and Null, Steve. *The New Vegetarian. Building Your Health Through Natural Eating.* New York: William Morrow & Co., 1978.

Padus, Emrika, and The Editors of Prevention Magazine. *A Complete Guide to Your Emotions and Your Health. New Dimensions in Body-Mind Healing.* Emmaus, PA: Rodale Press, 1986.

Shute, Wilfride, M.D., Health Preserver. *Defining the Versatility of Vitamin E.* Emmaus, PA: Rodale Press, 1977.

Williams, Roger J., Dr. *Nutrition Against Disease.* Huntington Beach, CA: International Institute of Natural Health Sciences.

ABOUT THE AUTHOR

For over 20 years, Trudy Lanitis has been involved in various forms of alternative healing as a serious student, teacher and healer.

Ms. Lanitis has appeared in training films on the subject of alternative healing, along with Dr. Patricia Heidt. Also, she has appeared in the book "The Heart of Healing" published by Turner Publishing in 1994. This book is based on the six-part TV series of the same name, produced by Turner Broadcasting.

She has developed her unique Bio-Etheric Healing method over the past six years to overcome the debilitating ailments of Lyme disease and rheumatoid arthritis.

Currently, Ms. Lanitis holds individual counseling sessions and conducts workshops in Bio-Etheric Healing for healing professionals and others interested in spiritual healing. Also, she provides individual instruction to professional healers, working towards developing a cadre of Bio-Etheric Healing professionals to spread this new found knowledge.

To further this work, she is teaching courses in Bio-Etheric Healing in various accredited institutions and colleges, and other learning centers with a focus on metaphysical studies. Most of her work takes place around St. Petersburg, Florida, and near her workspace in Kingston, New York.

Lord Kuthumi bestowed the honorary title of Master Healer on Trudy Lanitis in 1996.

To Learn More:
To find out more about Bio-Etheric Healing workshops, personalized teaching sessions, or individual healing consultations, write to:

Bio-Etheric Healing
c/o Trudy Lanitis
P.O. Box 58075
St. Petersburg, FL 33715

INDEX TO HEALINGS FOR SPECIFIC AILMENTS